Assessing health informatics and computing experiments

Keith Lui

Assessing health informatics and computing experiments

The Measurement of Informatics Controlled Experiments (MICE) index

VDM Verlag Dr. Müller

Impressum/Imprint (nur für Deutschland/ only for Germany)
Bibliografische Information der Deutschen Nationalbibliothek: Die Deutsche Nationalbibliothek
verzeichnet diese Publikation in der Deutschen Nationalbibliografie; detaillierte bibliografische
Daten sind im Internet über http://dnb.d-nb.de abrufbar.
 Alle in diesem Buch genannten Marken und Produktnamen unterliegen warenzeichen-, marken-
oder patentrechtlichem Schutz bzw. sind Warenzeichen oder eingetragene Warenzeichen der
jeweiligen Inhaber. Die Wiedergabe von Marken, Produktnamen, Gebrauchsnamen,
Handelsnamen, Warenbezeichnungen u.s.w. in diesem Werk berechtigt auch ohne besondere
Kennzeichnung nicht zu der Annahme, dass solche Namen im Sinne der Warenzeichen- und
Markenschutzgesetzgebung als frei zu betrachten wären und daher von jedermann benutzt
werden dürften.

Coverbild: www.purestockx.com

Verlag: VDM Verlag Dr. Müller Aktiengesellschaft & Co. KG
Dudweiler Landstr. 99, 66123 Saarbrücken, Deutschland
Telefon +49 681 9100-698, Telefax +49 681 9100-988, Email: info@vdm-verlag.de

Herstellung in Deutschland:
Schaltungsdienst Lange o.H.G., Berlin
Books on Demand GmbH, Norderstedt
Reha GmbH, Saarbrücken
Amazon Distribution GmbH, Leipzig
ISBN: 978-3-639-23354-4

Imprint (only for USA, GB)
Bibliographic information published by the Deutsche Nationalbibliothek: The Deutsche
Nationalbibliothek lists this publication in the Deutsche Nationalbibliografie; detailed
bibliographic data are available in the Internet at http://dnb.d-nb.de .
Any brand names and product names mentioned in this book are subject to trademark, brand or
patent protection and are trademarks or registered trademarks of their respective holders. The use
of brand names, product names, common names, trade names, product descriptions etc. even
without a particular marking in this works is in no way to be construed to mean that such names
may be regarded as unrestricted in respect of trademark and brand protection legislation and
could thus be used by anyone.

Cover image: www.purestockx.com

Publisher:
VDM Verlag Dr. Müller Aktiengesellschaft & Co. KG
Dudweiler Landstr. 99, 66123 Saarbrücken, Germany
Phone +49 681 9100-698, Fax +49 681 9100-988, Email: info@vdm-publishing.com

Printed in the U.S.A.
Printed in the U.K. by (see last page)
ISBN: 978-3-639-23354-4

Table of Contents

List of Tables

List of Figures and Boxes

6

Abbreviations

ACM: Association for Computing Machinery
AMIA: American Medical Informatics Association
ANOVA: analysis of variance
CASE: Computer-Assisted Software Engineering
CDSS: Clinical Decision Support System
CI: confidence interval
CPI: Consumer Price Index
CPU: Central Processing Unit
CTT: Classical Test Theory
df: degrees of freedom
EFMI: European Federation for Medical Informatics
H_0: null hypothesis
H_1/H_A: alternative hypothesis
HTML: Hypertext Markup Language
ICC: intraclass correlation coefficient
ICT: Information and Communications Technology
IEEE: Institute of Electrical and Electronics Engineers
IMRAD: Introduction, Method, Results And Discussion
INR: International Normalized Ratio
IS: Information Systems
ISCE: International Conference on Software Engineering
IT: Information Technology
JCR: Journal Citation Report
JIF: Journal Impact Factor
MeSH: Medical Subject Heading
MICE-38: Measurement of Informatics Controlled Experiments index with 38 items
MICE-80: Measurement of Informatics Controlled Experiments index with 80 items
NHMRC: National Health and Medical Research Council
PDA: Personal Data Assistant
UML: Unified Modeling Language

Chapter 1: Introduction

1.1.   General Introduction

The fields of computer science and health informatics present many questions. When a computer programmer asserts that placing Goto statements in code is bad, or when a health informatician states that a clinical information system prevents medical error, how are these known? Is a piece of paper with a decision algorithm as good as electronic decision support? Does computer-supported cooperative work actually improve work output? Do the benefits of computer technology outweigh the costs? How much information is needed to make good decisions in health care and other domains? As scholarly fields, computer science and health informatics must use rigorous research methods to answer such questions. Properly conducted research enables the determination of truth or falsity, and there are many paradigms and methods. One important paradigm is positivism, and one important method is the controlled experiment. Indeed, these 2 pillars represent the so-called "scientific method".

This book is an outcome of research into improving the quality of controlled experiments performed in computer science and health informatics. The quality of experimentation has been of concern to empirical scientists in both fields, which has lead to publication of textbooks and journal/conference papers on the subject to raise awareness and improve standards. However, if something is to be improved, it must undergo initial and ongoing assessment. Areas of deficiency must be identified and baseline observations made. Improvement is, by definition, comparative in nature. This research produces a measurement instrument, the Measurement of Informatics Controlled Experiments index or MICE index, to quantify experimental quality in health informatics and computer science. With this instrument, assessment and improvement can be achieved.

The example of the effects of a computer-based system on human performance outcomes is one area in which controlled experimentation can be useful. This is a form of summative evaluation. Experimentation can be useful in a formative sense also, e.g. to establish the best methods of constructing and maintaining software and to improve human-machine interfaces. Indeed, in a broad sense, experimentation facilitates the discovery of laws and principles that allow better development and use of computer-based technologies. However, there is more than one paradigm and one method of scholarly investigation. Qualitative methods can also yield knowledge in computer science and health informatics. The subjective impact of a new information system on a work group, for instance, may be measured better with qualitative, interpretivistic techniques. Similarly, understanding why people choose to use or not use computer technology or use only certain aspects may also be answered by non-experimental methods. The scope of evaluative and research methods that can be applied to computer science and health informatics is large. This book only focuses on improving controlled experimentation.

This chapter is divided into the following sections. Philosophical Background discusses how the research in this book fits with the fields of computer science and health informatics. To determine what is considered worthwhile research in these fields, the fields themselves must be examined. Research Motivation explains why this research was performed and how it addresses a significant current problem in informatics experimentation. Research Aims and Scope outlines the hypotheses and scope of the research. Research Method outlines the research paradigm and methods used. Contributions to Knowledge summarises how the fields of computer science and health informatics have been furthered. Finally, Book Overview explains the organisation of the rest of this book.

1.2. Philosophical Background

It is important to consider the philosophical basis for research in computer science and health informatics. For research in these fields to be considered original and contributing, there must be an examination of what exactly is the nature of the fields. Research in a field of study should follow the paradigms and practices of that field. For example, mathematics, physics and chemistry have well-defined ways of considering what is knowledge and how it is obtained. Therefore, research in these fields has an established framework to observe. The following section will demonstrate that the research and knowledge paradigms are far from trivial in computer science and health informatics.

The followed questions should be examined: what is computer science, what is health informatics and how do the two fields relate? Finally, how does this research fit with the paradigms in computer science and/or health informatics?

1.2.1. What is Computer Science?

The computer science literature has examined the nature of the field for 50 years without a consensus on what constitutes computer science (1). Hence this book, which does not focus specifically on this issue, is unlikely to provide a great leap forward. However, the question is implicitly visited every time a research dissertation, funding proposal or journal/conference submission is assessed for its worth, and so, some discussion is required. It will not be argued what computer science (or health informatics) should be but what perspectives exist and how they are related to research contribution. The term, "computer science", itself is subject to variable interpretation. It is conspicuous that Europeans use the term "informatics" while Americans use the term "computer science" (2). This issue of what is "informatics" will be revisited below. At the highest level, "computer science" can be used as an umbrella term for the various fields of study that involve computers, e.g. information technology (IT), information systems (IS), information and communications technology (ICT), software engineering, human-computer interaction, computer engineering but also includes related fields such as mathematics. On the other hand, the term can be interpreted as that specifically related to algorithms and modelling, without the necessity for (unnecessary and inelegant) implementation in any particular programming language (3). This is sometimes referred to as the distinction between computer science and computer engineering (4) (although even whether such a distinction should be made is debated (5)). That is, the former deals with theory of computation and the other with building engineering objects (such as software, computer hardware and information systems). The splintering of computer science (umbrella meaning) into differing subfields is noticeable in the literature, e.g. the process of establishing IT as a separate academic discipline under the Association for Computing Machinery (ACM) and the Institute of Electrical and Electronics Engineers (IEEE) (6), despite the "parent" field undergoing identity insecurity (this is also noticeable in health informatics as discussed later.) It is also mentionable that the subfields have also had difficulties with defining their area of research and practice, e.g. IS research (7-9) and human-computer interaction (10).

What is the definition of computer science? The ACM describes the computing discipline as incorporating computer engineering (design and construction of hardware), computer science (studies of ways to design and create software, to use computers and to solve computing problems), software engineering (studies of how better software can be created), information systems (use of computers to solve business information needs) and information technology (a technical focus of the use of computers for organisations) (11). Therefore, despite ideological differences, what is generally accepted is that computer science involves computers. As Denning et al note, the discipline was born in the 1940's with "the joining together of algorithm theory, mathematical logic, and the invention of the stored-program electronic computer." (4) This appears obvious, but some commentators have noted the dangers of defining a field based on a tool, as remarked by Dijkstra, "Computer science is not about computers, any more than astronomy is about telescopes," (3) (or surgery is about knives (12)). Then again, others have explicitly addressed the field as that which concentrates on computing tools (13). The idea of computer science necessarily involving computing technology appears ridiculously evident, but it is challenged when discussions turn to health informatics, as will be seen below.

One of the key features in the discussion of what is computer science is the distinction between science and engineering. This was described by Brooks as, "The scientist builds in order to study;

11

the engineer studies in order to build." (13) Research worthiness can be lost in such a distinction. To the scientist, who looks for generalisable, testable theories of computing, the mere construction of software and systems lacks research credibility. To the engineer, who looks for solutions to problems, the creation of a solution is perhaps sufficient. The latter idea may seem, to some, as intellectually barren, but it is present in computer science: the literature contains many demonstrations of computing artefacts. It is notable, in management IS research, that constructive research is promoted (this form of research from the fields of management and accounting credibly accepts the mere construction of solutions as long as they usefully solve a real-world problem (14).)

It is prudent to discuss what is meant by science in computer science. The issue of the scientific and/or engineering basis for computer science has been discussed in the literature for many years with many arguing that computer science should be more "scientific", e.g. (15-21). A report by the ACM Task Force on the Core of Computer Science described computer science as encompassing paradigms of theory, abstraction and design (4). Abstraction was noted to be "rooted in the experimental scientific method" and consisting of hypothesis formation and experimental design (4). This is the traditional interpretation of science: the formation of theories and universal knowledge or truths, and testing by repeatable empirical methods. Therefore, at least in some aspect of computer science, research must be more than mere creation of tools. However, Brooks and others, e.g. (22), argue the exact opposite, i.e. computer science is not science at all.

Returning to the question posed earlier, what is computer science, the above discussion shows that different views exist:

- Computer science is (or should be) science, in the traditional sense of science, e.g. (15, 20)

- Computer science is engineering, e.g. (13).

- Computer science is a blend of science and engineering (and other areas), e.g. (3, 5).

Whether the research in this book contributes to computer science is discussed below.

1.2.2.   What is Health Informatics?

The literature in computer science demonstrates a lack of consensus for the field in terms of philosophical underpinning. Unfortunately, health informatics fares less well and is further complicated by the addition of health science paradigms. Before elaborating on health informatics, it is useful to consider what is the difference, if any, between "informatics" and "computer science". As mentioned above, the two may be considered synonyms in parts of Europe. Historically, informatics indeed meant computer science. It was first coined by the German father of computer science, Karl Steinbuch, in his 1957 paper (Informatik: automatische informationsverbeitung) and became the German term for computer science (23). In 1962, the French computer scientist, Philippe Dreyfus, used the term "informatique" (24), and its meaning, to this day, is computer science. It was in 1966/67 that the Russian information scientist, Mikhailov, used "informatika" to mean the field concerning the properties and structure of information (with respect to scientific information) (24). Today, the meaning of informatics can be thought of as the field that combines information science with computer science and involves individual, societal and computational processing of information. However, some still suggest that informatics is closer to computer science than information science (or other related fields), e.g. Buerk and Feig state, "People are recognizing informatics as a subdiscipline within computer science education..." and, "One area of IT... is the field of informatics." (25) The historical roots of health informatics, or medical informatics as it was known then, are similar to general informatics. Also in the sixties, German university departments of medical informatics were being created and were among the first in the world (26). At that time, health (medical) informatics indeed meant the application of computer science to medicine (26). From the perspective given thus far, it might be reasonable that, based on taxonomy, informatics is a computing field. Therefore, health informatics is a computing field (the application of informatics to health care).

1.2.3. Divisions in Health Informatics

Unfortunately, the concept of health informatics has not remained simply as computer science in medicine. Much has been written over the last 40 years about what is health informatics, and, like computer science, there are divisions. Before progressing further, it is useful to clarify the meaning of "health" and "medical". Health refers to all aspects of health care, e.g. provision of care by health workers including doctors, nurses, dentists, physiotherapists and so on, as well as the structures of health care services. "Medical" can be synonymous with "health" in this sense. Another interpretation of "medical" is as an adjective referring to doctors (therefore "medical informatics" would refer to informatics in the work of doctors). In this book, no distinction is made between "health" and "medical", though this is not always the case in the health/medical informatics community.

Perspectives of health informatics are complicated by the field's youth. The true pioneers (those with no formal training in health informatics) still contribute to the research agenda. Even the second generation scholars likely have one area of primary discipline supplemented by another, e.g. computer professional plus extra health training or health professional with extra computing training (27). Researchers in the field have come from a variety of backgrounds: computer science, engineering, information science, health care, librarianship, business and management, sociology and others. These people have brought with them the epistemology of their background fields. Anecdotally, many of the early scholars in health informatics were (and still are) medical practitioners. The health informatics literature reveals the desire of this clinical group of health informaticians to make health informatics a part of medicine, rather than computer science. Blois proposed that health informatics was a science to improve the understanding of medicine, that it could help model the knowledge of medicine, and therefore the two are intrinsically related (28). Such an inextricable bond was also suggested by Detmer (29). Some have proposed that health informaticians should also be practising clinicians (30). Hasman called health informatics a distinct, separate discipline but also that it "forms one of the bases of medicine and health care." (31) One of strongest proponents of the idea that health informatics is more medicine than computing has been Reinhold Haux, current president of the International Medical Informatics Association (32):

Medical informatics is not just the application of computers in medicine and health care. (33)

Medical informatics is a scientific medical discipline, like surgery or internal medicine, like epidemiology or microbiology. It is a medical discipline with strong relationships to the health sciences concerning the field of application and with strong relationships to informatics concerning its methods and tools. (33)

We should obviously concentrate our work on the medical problem under investigation and not, as in computer science, on the tool 'computer' or on methods for this tool. (34)

As an example of this ideology, he suggested that research into electronic medical records must also include research into the regular patient record, independent of the computer tool (33). That is, what are the models behind the recording and content of patient data (35), irrespective of computerisation?

Other clinically based informaticians have voiced similar ideas:

Most people equate medical informatics with computers, which is logical enough, but we think the field should be considered in a much broader way, as the science of information and communication related to medical care, whether or not computers are involved. (36)

I have now broadened the scope of our discipline from computer disciplines applied to medicine to the concept of medical information disciplines... It is intellectually improper to build a discipline on the application of a given tool (computing machinery), whatever its complexity and its historical importance. (37)

We will need people who are knowledge engineers rather than computer scientists. (38)

These ideas are similarly held by some medical societies, e.g. the European Society of Intensive Care Medicine's position on health informatics is that it is "not tied to the application of computers but more generally to the entire management of information in healthcare." (39)

The idea of medical ownership of health informatics has been taken even further with each specialist group in health care calling for their own share, e.g. "The unique nature of primary care necessitates the development of its own informatics discipline," argued De Lusignan in favour of establishing primary care informatics (40).

Haynes et al's statement (36) that computers may or may not be involved is a key distinction often made by clinically based informaticians. This is the view that health informatics is an information modelling field where computer technology can be of assistance. However, there may be other forms of improving the quality of information in medicine, e.g. paper-based clinical algorithms. Therefore, computing is often required but not necessary in thinking about what health informatics is. Even the work that initially started under medical computer science in Germany was directed down a medical information science path as the "synthesis of information processes." (26) This is not to say this perspective of health informatics regards computer science as unimportant. Indeed, health informatics has been criticised by some of these proponents for failing to use methods successful in computer science (41), instead reinventing an inferior wheel. While the tools might be shared, the focus between computer science and health informatics is different. The focus is not the development of the computer for health care but how better information can benefit the patient. As Imhoff reminded, "Without patients there would be no need for health informatics." (39)

With this clinical perspective of health informatics in mind, it is remarkable to contrast it against the computing perspective. In 1977, an ACM subcommittee was established by the ACM Education Board to develop a curriculum for the "health computing professional" (42, 43). Four tracks were identified: health information systems, health research computing, computer-based health education and health computing administration. As with the definition of computer science previously stated, it makes little sense to discuss any of these tracks without the presence of a computer. The focus on the computer in health informatics has continued through to today (25, 44-46). This is in direct contrast to the above clinical views of health informatics. Karen Duncan, who was part of the ACM subcommittee in 1977, implored clinicians to take more leadership in health computing or for the scope of medical informatics to be "alternatively defined so that others may lead the way." (45) Ironically, it has been the very involvement of some clinically based health informaticians that has contributed to divisions in the field.

15

One can observe the different stakeholders that wish to shape health informatics, by examining the evolution of professional societies. Health informatics groups have developed in parallel to health computing groups. Ironically, some of these health informatics associations began as subgroups under computing groups, e.g. the Health Informatics Society of Australia (which began under the Australian Computer Society) (47) and the International Medical Informatics Association (which began under the International Federation for Information Processing) (48). On the computing side, some of the ACM Special Interest Groups have interest in biological and health-related computing (49). On the (biomedical) engineering side, there is the IEEE Engineering in Medicine and Biology Society, which covers a wide range of technical interests, including prosthetics, medical devices, medical imaging and information systems (50). One of the reasons for the separation of health informatics groups was the influence of clinical medicine. Some early clinical pioneers moved health informatics away from computer science and technology, and this shaped the political and research landscape.

In addition to separation of professional groups, background has influenced research publication. Computer scientists prefer conference publications (51), whereas the tradition in medicine has been prestigious journals (e.g. the Lancet). Medicine also influences publishing conventions, with journals such as the International Journal of Medical Informatics (official journal of the European Federation for Medical Informatics) and the Journal of the American Medical Informatics Association endorsing the International Committee of Medical Journal Editors (ICMJE) standards (52, 53). Why not ACM standards? When indexing health informatics literature, should the U.S. National Library of Medicine's Medical Subject Heading (MeSH) terms be used or the IEEE Computer Society's keywords?

Another example of biomedicine's influence, that is particularly relevant to this book, is in evaluation frameworks for information systems. The Declaration of Innsbruck provides a framework for health information system evaluation and was produced by an EFMI working group. However, it developed from a workshop meeting of mostly health (informatics) scientists (54). Should evaluation of information systems be focused at the health care level or more generally? If health researchers do not work with computing researchers, then evaluation theories and methods might be unnecessarily duplicated. It is not inconceivable that IS evaluation researchers have not at all heard of the declaration. A search of the ACM Digital Library, an often-used bibliographical database in computer science, reveals no reference to the declaration outside of one paper (in the Journal of Biomedical Informatics), and no results arise for the IEEE Xplore database (also well-used).

Despite the strong influence of medicine, the issue of where health informatics should lie is not resolved. So far the focus of this discussion has been on the two main pillars of health informatics: medicine and computer science. However, there are other component disciplines, e.g. Perry et al argued that medical informatics is similar to medical librarianship (55). Whetton recently wrote about the divergent nature of health informatics (56). She called for a dialogue to form between factions in health informatics to combat the divergence but also called for more social research to be part of health informatics. The large number of paradigms and methods add to the confusion of a core for health informatics.

In summary, some, like for computer science, argue that health informatics is engineering, e.g. (57). Some argue that health informatics is a (medical) discipline in its own right, with its own body of scientific knowledge and methods, e.g. (58-61). Some believe that health informatics is a branch of applied computer science, e.g. (46, 62). Others believe that health informatics is a basic science for the larger fields in health care, e.g. (63). The fable of the blind men and the elephant is poignant at this time in health informatics' evolution. Each blind man is holding a different part of the animal: the biomedical engineer touching its side and claiming a wall, the physician holding onto the tail and claiming a rope, the business manager holding onto the leg and claiming a tree, the medical librarian holding onto the tusk and claiming a spear and the computing professional holding onto the ear and claiming a fan. With computing and communications technology ever advancing, and increasing dependence of health care processes on this technology, perhaps the future of health informatics will return to its origin and become more solidified in computer science. However, with health informatics programmes that direct the field away from computer science, such as the well-established ones at the University of Heidelberg/School of Technology Heilbronn (which promotes that the field is "more than a discipline just based on methods and tools of informatics applied to medicine and health care" (64)) and at the University of Amsterdam (which treats its curriculum as "medical study, meaning that computer science is rather positioned as one of the auxiliary sciences…" (65)), the future of where health informatics sits is likely to remain contested.

1.2.4. The Effects of Background on Health Informatics

There are 2 related effects of the influence of medicine on health informatics: the scientific tradition and evidence-based evaluation. Medicine is a strongly positivistic, scientifically oriented discipline. Its influence has lead to many calls for seeking the scientific theories underlying health informatics (31, 37, 59, 61, 66, 67) and criticism towards publication of merely descriptive reports of information systems and other computer-based tools that do not provide scientific insight (41, 66). There are numerous recommendations for health informatics products, e.g. clinical decision support systems, to be evaluated for their effects on patients, health care providers, organisations etc, e.g.

(31, 39, 68-73). Clinicians are very conscious of evidence-based medical practice (74), which gives rise to comments such as:

For a system to be worth while, it should be based on evidence that implementation of the reminder system is more likely to do good than harm. Unfortunately, most system developers haven't a clue about what solid health care evidence is. (36)

Evidence-based practice has not been as prominent in computer science (e.g. advocacy research) as it has been in medicine (75, 76), which is hardly surprising since computer science is not medicine. However, health informatics gets caught in the middle. Shortliffe wrote the following, which reflects the influence of medical science and university departments on the scientific orientation in health informatics:

I also remember encountering serious questions (and condescending attitudes) from fellow academicians who worked at our medical school in more traditional fields of research. Somehow medical informatics did not seem to be 'real science' to them, and this forced me to consider how best to create and promote a research and training program in informatics so that it would gain credibility and peer respect. (77)

Shortliffe's thoughts are noteworthy because they suggest that health informatics research in the setting of a medical faculty should adhere to a standard of medical science research. Would health informatics research in a computing faculty be expected to conform likewise?

One of the best examples of how medical science has influenced health informatics is the topic of controlled experimentation. Because of the scientific and evidence-based approaches from medicine, controlled experimentation (or controlled trials) in health informatics has been encouraged by many (60, 63, 67, 68, 78, 79).

However, it would be incorrect to state that evaluation and controlled experimental evaluation in health informatics is universally agreed upon. Rather, the traditions of medical research have pushed health informatics further into experimentation than has occurred in computer science. By contrast, mathematics historically had a strong influence on computer science and brought a tradition of mathematical proof (4, 21). This is despite significant experimental work in computer programming that occurred in the late 1960's and 1970's (80).

1.2.5. The Importance of Philosophical Background

Are the underpinnings of computer science and health informatics actually important? In the opinion of the author, the answer is yes. The discussion about where computer science and health

18

informatics sit in terms of underlying principles is not just important for how research practice should be viewed. It has implication in funding, teaching, publication acceptability, organisation of university departments, career advancement and professional and discipline identity.

With respect to funding, should money be given to computer science departments, medical departments or health informatics departments (or others)? A good example of where competition for limited funds might occur is the lucrative field of biological computing (bioinformatics) in the era of the human genome (81). The computer is essential in bioinformatics, and it is noteworthy that bioinformatics has been recognised formally as an applied area of computer science (11). Yet, others wish to incorporate bioinformatics as part of health informatics, hence the emerging term "biomedical informatics" (82). By positioning an area of study under a specific discipline, the area may gain recognition as being owned by the parent, and funding flows accordingly.

With respect to departmental arrangements, Huang recently examined programmes in health informatics around the world and noted that departments outside of health science are also placing their stamp on the field, i.e. masters degrees in business administration and commerce with specialisation in health informatics have arisen (83). Is it acceptable for any department that contributes an area of knowledge to health informatics to establish their own flavour of the field? Such notions would impact upon what education is offered and by which university departments.

With respect to teaching, the issue of what is the core of a field becomes readily apparent because decisions must be made on what is incorporated into a programme and what is not. It is noteworthy that a health informatics curriculum (46) established by a computer science department and focusing on teaching computer science students (rather than health students) fails to address experimental evaluation. Johnson similarly noted the issue: "Computer science is less interested in empirical methods. Experimental design is not a component of most computer science curricula..." (67)

In terms of health informatics research worthiness, Reinhold Haux was direct:

If research in medical informatics means scientific research we should concentrate on methodology not application of a certain tool. We should concentrate on medical informatics, not on biomedical computing... It has considerable consequences for the orientation of research and education in medical informatics. (33)

Medical informatics is not just a mixture of fields of medicine and informatics... research with methods and tools from the field of informatics − even when medical examples are taken −

19

without specific orientation to research questions in medicine and health care is, as such, no medical informatics research. (33)

Their interpretation of health informatics research indicates that computer science and health informatics research would be separate. For example, a computing algorithm useful in both medicine and another domain (such as banking) might be a worthy research outcome in computer science but not according to Haux's requirement. A narrow view of research prevents the problem of, as Detmer put it, "When anything goes, anything grows," (29) but stifles potentially significant research before it has begun.

Another view of worthy health informatics research was put forward in Shortliffe and Cimino's text:

A dissertation worthy of a PhD in the field will usually be identified by a generalizable scientific result that also contributes to one of the component disciplines and on which other scientists can build in the future. (82) (p. 37)

This model identifies computer science as one of several components and opposes the ideas of Haux, suggesting that computer science and health informatics research are not separate.

1.2.6.   Philosophical Implications for this Book

The discussions so far have been important in understanding whether the author's research fits with the paradigms of computer science and health informatics. Both fields are characterised by multiple views of what they are and how research and other scholarly activities should be conducted. Other fields influence both and can lay claim to knowledge ownership. Quantitative, qualitative, positivistic, interpretivistic, empirical and non-empirical research paradigms exist. Evaluation and controlled experimentation is viewed as both essential and not so essential. It is no wonder, even after 40 to 50 years, that commentators regard both fields as suffering from identity crises. Maojo even argued that health informatics does not have an established paradigm yet and is, from a Kuhnian perspective, prescience (84).

Perhaps one solution to this problem is to accept that the fields, at this point in history, are pluralistic and multidisciplinary. Such a view is workable in health research, e.g. research in the field of public health. Research can then follow a paradigm (and method) that is acceptable to the fields, as long as the tenets are upheld and the paradigm continues to provide answers. The scientific paradigm, evaluation perspective and the experimental method have all been areas of research in both computer science and health informatics. Research may be seen as a journey down one of several paths of pluralism and justified on this basis. Furthermore, to research experimental methods is to not deny qualitative ones or mathematical ones.

Another view is a return to basic principles. Assuming that science is accepted as a foundation for computer science and health informatics, then research that contributes to basic science would be important to the fields. A basic science project may contribute to underlying principles and might be considered superior to mere development of computing artefacts. The author's research asserts that controlled experimentation is part of basic scientific research. Therefore, the improvement of experimental quality in computer science and health informatics would be contributory research. In other words, research that improves the acquisition of knowledge is inherently worthwhile.

From a health informatics versus computer science perspective, whether or not research should keep to one or both will probably remain a point of contention. This research was based on both domains and can be applied to both, which is consistent with Shortliffe and Cimino's view above but will attract criticism from those who view health informatics as its own discipline. Indeed, health informatics evaluation appears to be studied with little reference to general computing evaluation. Nevertheless, research that spans disciplines may be important for unifying computer science and health informatics.

Returning to the final question, does this research fit with the paradigms of computer science and health informatics, it is argued that it does. It addresses a fundamental basic science issue shared by both fields and follows the tenets of the scientific paradigm, which has a distinct role in both.

1.3.   Research Motivation

This research is motivated by deficiencies of knowledge in both health informatics and computer science. From the previous discussion of philosophical background, it can be seen that research in one is possible without consideration of the other. Health informatics and computer science can and have developed identities and research outcomes at different pace, whether they be computing artefacts or controlled experimentation. Ignorance of each other's developments ultimately adds to divergence, with each field possibly reinventing each other's wheels. If good experimentation conduct can improve the development of and establish principles for computer and information-based artefacts in both general informatics and health informatics, then reinvention of quality improvement methods would be wasteful. Therefore, this research adopted the approach as suggested by Shortliffe (82), i.e. research should contribute to a component discipline in addition to health informatics. This work provides a unified view of controlled experimentation in informatics research.

21

1.3.1. Improving Science, Experimentation and Evaluation

This research is motivated by deficiencies in scientific foundation and scientific evaluation. There is a close relationship between evaluation, experimentation and science. Technology evaluation can occur for several reasons, including feedback of results to inform scientific development of future tools. The importance of evaluation has been recognised in some areas of computer science, e.g. case study research in management information systems (85) (as well as other qualitative type research (86)) and empirical software engineering (17, 87, 88). An evaluative mindset distinguishes craft or trade from science. The craftsman is satisfied if an object meets its required specifications. The scientist, however, is further intrigued by how to improve the object and must somehow evaluate the object or the ways in which it was made. The empirical scientist will use formal methods, such as the controlled experiment. It is common to see the triad of concepts arise in computing research, whether health or otherwise, where investigators wonder whether the building of objects without some rigorous experimental evaluation to learn something more is acceptable. Holloway, for example, wrote:

> This ignorance manifests itself in the plethora of people who jump on the latest-and-greatest 'methodology' bandwagon (functional decomposition, rapid prototyping, object orientation, CASE tools, reuse techniques, and process maturity are just a few such bandwagons) on the basis of 'success stories' and slick sales pitches. The notion of requesting actual logical or experimental evidence of success seems not to enter the picture. (89)

Tierney et al (78) called for controlled trials of health informatics applications to, among other reasons, understand what are the additional information gains from better technology and whether they could be achieved with simpler solutions. They, like Holloway, also spoke of experimental summative evaluation of technology and the importance of a scientific mindset.

The influence of medical science on the development of a triad of evaluation, experimentation and science in health informatics can be seen from the above sections. In computer science, experimentation has historically not had a large place in computing knowledge. In 1995, Tichy et al found that about half of the 400 research articles they reviewed lacked adequate experimental validation (90). Similar results were found by Zelkowitz el al around the same time (19). More recently, a review of software engineering scientific papers from 1993 to 2002 found that only 103 of 5453 (1.9%) reports were of controlled experiments (91). However, there are many researchers who are promoting experimental methods in computer science (17-19, 76, 88, 92-95). This is especially in the subdiscipline of software engineering, which has a journal (Empirical Software Engineering) and conference (Empirical Software Engineering and Measurement) dedicated to experimentation and other empirical methods. Change is also occurring at the level of the undergraduate computer science curriculum to include experimental design and statistical analysis (96, 97), which have historically been ignored in computer science education (16). Empirical and experimental research is likely to grow in computer science as researchers become more aware of the dangers of advocacy research and the limitations of other research methods in answering certain questions, such as subtle summative effects of information technologies. This is not to say that other forms of knowledge discovery are unimportant. Indeed, experimentation would be inappropriate in situations where mathematical proof or qualitative interview can better answer a question. Ideally, all research methods in computer science (and health informatics) should be used with high quality assurance, and attempts may be made to raise standards comprehensively, but that is beyond the scope of this research.

1.3.2. Problems in Experimental Quality

While experimentation is an important method in health informatics and increasingly important in computer science, there have been concerns that quality should be improved in both fields. Tierney et al lamented the short supply of researchers who understand both health informatics and controlled experimentation and called for further funding and training (78). Dimitroff analysed health informatics research papers and found several problems, including inadequately defined variables and hypotheses and poor integration of findings with previous knowledge. Others have also noted experimental mistakes such as unit of analysis error (98), contamination effects and other biases (99). The Declaration of Innsbruck, though recommending at the level of general evaluation of health information systems, calls for high standards of scientific evaluation methods (which would include experimentation) (54). Chapter 5 reviews the quality of experiments for clinical decision support systems and highlights some of these methodological problems. As for computer science experimentation, the inadequacy of experimental education has been noted. One of the manifestations of this deficiency has been poor quality of experiments. Moher and Schneider at the International Conference on Software Engineering (ICSE) of 1981 discussed the issue of experimental rigor, stating, "While there are numerous references to the use of experimentation there are significantly fewer references to the methodology itself." (100) Problems with performing reliable and valid experiments due to poor methodology still occur despite Moher's warning. In the ICSE of 2006, Zannier et al presented findings of their review of ICSE papers (101), stating "The soundness of empirical evaluations has not improved over 29 years of ICSE proceedings," and "Except for one study in our random sample, none of the examined studies contained hypotheses clearly stated." Another manifestation is the adequacy of reviewers of computer science experiments: "Papers about empirical work in software engineering are still somewhat of a novelty

23

and reviewers, especially those inexperienced with empirical work themselves, are often unsure whether a paper is good enough for publication." (102)

Ultimately, the problem with poor experimentation is that it can lead to dissemination of incorrect knowledge. This is particularly problematic for health informatics experiments, when safety-critical technologies are evaluated. Poor experimental results may misleadingly support or deny the adoption of technologies to patients' detriment.

1.3.3.   Quality Assurance: Guidelines and Scales

Efforts are being made to improve experimental quality in computer science and health informatics. One way has been to publish guidelines and standards in the literature. Another way, which is the focus of this research, is to measure quality with scales or indexes. Chapter 2 and Chapter 3 further discuss scales and the literature on experimental guidelines respectively. Why is it necessary to use measurement instruments such as scales and indexes to quantify quality? Could peer review be just as adequate? The insufficient number of reviewers educated in informatics and experimentation suggests otherwise. Moreover, peer review is itself a form of measurement. Unlike peer review, formal measurement of quality explicitly addresses reliability and validity. If studies are required to be assessed by referees, then it is only logical that the process is accurate.

Health informatics and computer science face similar challenges in experimentation as medical science. Medical controlled experimentation serves as a good example for quality assurance (irrespective of health informatics ties to medicine) and demonstrates why formal measurement is necessary for informatics experiments. The controlled experiment in medicine is regarded as the most rigorous form of evidence and afforded the highest level of credibility. This is internationally recognised in the form of "levels of evidence" frameworks, with systematic reviews of controlled trials at the top and less rigorous methods below, e.g. observational studies, uncontrolled studies and expert opinion. Australia's National Health and Medical Research Council (103), the U.S. Preventive Services Task Force and the U.K. National Health Service (104) endorse this model of evidence credibility. Medical controlled trials are important, but researchers have been concerned that quality is substandard, even to this day (105-107). This occurs despite many controlled trials, great effort, manpower, funding and many journals dedicated to trials and biostatistics. Why should controlled trials be performed well? Firstly, they hold great weight. There is esteem associated with controlled experiments that confers believability of the results, which go on to influence patient care. Secondly, they are resource intensive involving human participants, time and money. Thirdly, there is an ethical responsibility to those who participate. To address quality problems, guidelines and scales have been developed. The most well-known guideline is the Consolidated Standards Of

Reporting Trials (CONSORT) (108), which is endorsed by the ICMJE, and is thus the standard for many biomedical journals. It requires investigators to complete a checklist of common experimental quality issues before a study may be published. Scales have also been developed to measure controlled clinical trial quality. Guidelines and scales are quite established for medical trials. In 1995, Moher et al published an often-cited review of 25 scales and 9 checklists (109). In 2001, Verhagen et al estimated the number of scales to be between 50 and 60 (110). These instruments quantify clinical trial quality, and there is empirical evidence that applying a structured assessment does lead to improvement in quality (111).

Computer science and health informatics experimentation would benefit from following the example of clinical trial quality assurance. If medicine, with a large exposure to experiments, seeks to improve quality, then other experimental sciences should pay attention. This is particularly pertinent to health informatics, if it is to be viewed as a "medical discipline". Furthermore, clinical trials of health computing tools and their effects on patients and health care providers are increasingly commonplace (112). As argued in Chapter 3, adequate scales for measuring the quality of controlled experiments in computer science and health informatics are lacking. The primary motivation for this research was to address this gap and produce a tested scale. This research may be ahead of its time for computer science since experimental evaluation is not yet a mainstay of research and guidelines are still in their early stages. Jedlitschka et al (113) commented that the first published guideline for the reporting of computing experiments was as recent as 1999 (114). However, if the example of medicine is followed further, as has been quoted in the computer science literature (76), attention will eventually turn from developing guidelines to assessing quality.

1.3.4. Should Experimentation be a Focus? What about other Methods?

While experimentation has been argued above to have an important role in computer science and health informatics research, it is not without opposition in both fields and indeed even in medicine. Moehr argued that controlled trials in health informatics cannot accommodate the dynamically changing nature of information systems (115). Indeed, the focus on quantitative approaches has been challenged in favour of qualitative ones (116, 117). Tichy provided some reasons why computer scientists oppose experimentation, such as demonstrations being sufficient as proof (18). In health care, McManus offered a similar view that controlled trials should not be the gold standard for ensuring quality, giving the example of how products of engineering (e.g. aeroplanes) are constructed based on "theories and experience" (118). In other words, in engineering at least, if theory is sufficient to construct objects, then the construction of such objects is adequate scientific proof.

The essence of all research methods is their ability to make accurate and confident prediction. In a sense, McManus' view is correct. If adequate blueprints of a phenomenon exist, which can predict with confidence outcomes before they occur, then analysis, experimental or otherwise, may not be necessary. For example, it can be confidently demonstrated that binary search algorithms of sorted lists are logarithmic in time, based on an understanding of mathematics. When human beings are involved, predicting phenomena becomes more challenging. How confidently do research methods predict how humans and information resources/computers interact? Experimentation is merely one method to formulate accurate predictions, but it does it well. When done properly, it has rigor, meaning that sources of error (or untruth) affect prediction accuracy less than other methods, all things being equal. Phenomena are often subtle when studying humans, and rigor helps to identify real effects from other explanations. One should ask: how much confidence is inherent in a method for a particular research question, and how much confidence is required to make decisions and policies about informatics technologies and processes? Non-experimental methods may well suffice.

It is unfortunate that disagreement over research methods occurs. Experiments have their place, and arguments in favour of controlled experiments above other methods or for other methods over experimentation should be avoided. Strengths and weaknesses can be complementary. What is more important is that methods are performed to high standards. This research has focussed on controlled experimental quality. Other research might seek to improve qualitative methods. All are worthy since improving research quality improves confidence of prediction.

1.4. Research Aims and Scope

The previous section on Research Motivation raised a pivotal issue; the quality of controlled experiments in informatics involving human participants is largely ad-hoc, largely incomplete, and mechanisms to support quality is an open area for research. This issue formed the context for the establishment of the first hypothesis. Two broad areas were highlighted as considered within health informatics involving human participants, namely computer science and health informatics, and hence lead to the creation of the second and third hypotheses. Therefore, the primary hypotheses for this research were that:

- A questionnaire instrument that could measure the quality of controlled experiments could be defined for experiments in informatics involving human participants.

- The questionnaire instrument as proposed in hypothesis 1 can be applied within the domain of computer science.

- The questionnaire instrument as proposed in hypothesis 1 can be applied within the domain of health informatics.

In support of these hypotheses, the practical use of the instrument was demonstrated via applying it to a set of controlled experiments of clinical decision support systems, which is a common area for experimentation to be applied.

The scope of this research was limited to experimentation in informatics that involves human participants. In principle, controlled experiments can be applied to other aspects of computing, e.g. hardware design and performance. However, the more interesting experiments involve humans. Informatics is a human-centred activity. Without humans, there would be no need for information processing or the development of tools to aid information processing. The subtle interaction between information resources, computers and humans requires careful empirical methods because particular sources of error and confounding arise when studying humans, e.g. expectation and learning effects. As Weinberg noted in his aptly named text, "The Psychology of Computer Programming" (119), and in (120), human variability makes for challenging and important research.

This research should not be confused with one that might focus on evaluation. There has been much written about evaluation in computer science and health informatics, and this research does not attempt to cover the body of knowledge. This research does not aim to improve all evaluation methods or provide an overarching evaluation framework for computer science and health informatics (such as the Declaration of Innsbruck (54)). Guidelines of evaluation are important, but evaluation is only as useful as the proper conduct of underlying methods. In this research, only the experimental method is given attention. Moreover, while evaluation and experimentation (or other methods, e.g. qualitative) are closely related, their purposes may differ. Experimentation is a useful technique to develop scientific theory, but further developing scientific theory may not be a goal of a particular evaluation exercise. Stakeholders in evaluation may have concerns other than scientific theory. Therefore, improving a research method is not necessarily synonymous with improving evaluation.

1.5. Research Method

The outline of the research is shown in Chapter 3, Figure 2 and is explained in detail in Chapter 3. The literature on experimental guidelines and particularly on quality measurement instruments was examined from three fields: computer science, health informatics and medicine. After a semi-quantitative analysis of the literature, experimental concepts were identified and pooled, and a questionnaire was developed using psychometric principles. These principles are explained further

27

in Chapter 2. The questionnaire was assessed for its reliability and validity in measuring experimental quality and underwent further refinement to improve efficiency.

This research strongly drew upon positivism and measurement principles. Several assumptions are made in this research:

- Quality can be defined, measured and subjected to statistical analysis.

- Measurement should be precise, accurate and repeatable.

- Hypothesis testing around concepts of quality is possible.

This research is also constructivist in nature; a tool has been constructed that solves a practical problem. The questionnaire measures and improves the problem of experimental quality in informatics.

Other fields of study were referred to in the conduct of this research. Measurement of the obscure has been the forte of psychometrics for over 100 years (121), and quality is indeed an obscure phenomenon. Health informatics and computer science have not developed theories of measurement that can be used to quantify experimental quality as usefully as those from psychometrics. As for referring to medical trial quality scores and guidelines, there is a relatively large body of knowledge that may inform experimental practice in health informatics and computer science. Potentially, other experimental fields could be used, but there are reasons that medicine is useful. Firstly, there is the close relationship between health informatics and medicine. Secondly, medicine as an exemplary field is as good as any, given its experience with experimentation and quality assurance. Thirdly, the comparison of medicine has already been made in the computer science literature (122, 123). By referring to other experimental fields (another example is psychology (114)), informatics experimentation and quality improvement can avoid pitfalls and reinvention of wheels.

1.6.   Contributions to Knowledge

This research has demonstrated the hypotheses of producing a tested score for measuring experimental quality in informatics. The instrument can be used to quantify baseline quality and address areas for improvement. While quality improvement and quantification has been studied in other experimental fields, this has yet to be achieved in computer science and to an adequate degree in health informatics. The contribution is important because basic research quality is critical to scientific knowledge. Good experimentation may also be beneficial to deciding whether health informatics and computer science have satisfactory scientific foundations and is, therefore, important from a discipline point of view.

Quality is a difficult construct to understand. What is quality and how should we measure it? This is no trivial subject, as Robert Pirsig famously wrote about (124). Defining and measuring vague constructs when they are poorly understood is as important as the actual measurement process. This research makes an important contribution in examining experimental quality by producing quantitative evidence of the theoretical behaviour of quality in informatics experiments. For example, it was found that other indicators of research quality (Journal Impact Factor, The Thompson Corporation, Stamford, USA) do not correlate well with experimental quality. Research into developing quality measurement instruments for informatics experiments is only at the beginning. Lord Kelvin said, "To measure is to know," but to know how to measure is even more important. This means that methods to measure quality still need development and thought. This research is not only important for developing an instrument but also for contributing to the methodology of measuring quality.

Applying the MICE index to experimental evaluation of clinical decision support systems also contributes to knowledge in health informatics. A current review of the quality of controlled trials of clinical decision support systems is the product of this effort. This is an important step in monitoring the quality of research that leads to decision making about health technologies.

Indirectly, there have been other contributions to computer science and health informatics in the conduct of this research. By examining experimentation in health informatics, one must consider to what extent knowledge is shared by its component disciplines. Experimentation in health informatics and computer science can exist in isolation, but this situation is dangerous. Would it be acceptable for computerisation methods in health informatics and computer science to develop in isolation? This research tries to bridge the gap between the fields in the context of experimentation, and that is an original and important contribution. This research raises questions for further research with regards to how research should be reconciled in health (or any field of) informatics and computer science.

As a result of this work, the author has created a tool that can be integrated as part of the research process for future research within the domains of computer science and health informatics.

1.7. Book Overview

This book is organised into six main chapters. This chapter dealt with the background of philosophy and motivation and explained how this research fits in the fields of computer science and health informatics. Chapter 2 provides a general review of psychometric theory and scale construction in order to explain the principles of developing the MICE index. Chapter 3 describes the process of developing the MICE index, including initial literature search, questionnaire creation and reliability and validity testing. Chapter 4 produces and explains the questionnaire items, i.e. why items are important and how they should be interpreted and scored. Chapter 5 is a review of recent controlled trials of clinical decision support tools and demonstrates a use for the MICE index. It also provides further validation data for the testing procedures adopted in Chapter 3. The final chapter, six, concludes by summarising the results of this research. It also discusses strengths and limitations and what future work is needed.

Chapter 2: Introduction to Measurement and Scales

2.1.   Introduction

Chapter 1 explained the multiple paradigms and research methods available to informatics scientists. It also explained the positivistic, measurement-oriented basis for this research and the need to be multidisciplinary, borrowing methods from other quantitative fields. This chapter deals with realising the quantitative approach, using methods that have been developed and applied in other scientific disciplines. Most importantly, this chapter demonstrates some of the knowledge required for demonstrating the first hypothesis of this research: developing a reliable and valid quality instrument for human-based informatics controlled experiments. This chapter also shows how scale theory can be applied to support the second and third hypotheses: scales developed for computer science and health informatics experiments. Much of the science behind quantitative research has been established in fields such as psychology, sociology and education. However, the measurement of experimental quality in informatics demonstrates deficiencies that this research has addressed. In that sense, this research also contributes to psychometric evaluation as applied to informatics experimentation. These contributions are discussed in Chapter 3.

This chapter describes the general principles of measurement and scale development, since it is acknowledged that psychometric methods are not often part of the armamentarium of skills and knowledge possessed by informatics researchers. In particular, how these methods are used to measure experimental quality is even less known by informaticians. However, this chapter is not intended to be at all comprehensive of psychometric methods, as there are textbooks dedicated to them but rather to highlight concepts important to the author's research.

At this point, a caution regarding the use of the term "scale" should be made. In addition to a synonym for level of measurement, scale can refer to a type of measurement instrument and the responses of a questionnaire item. All of these concepts are discussed further in this chapter.

2.2.   Importance of Measurement

The physicist, Lord Kelvin, said of measurement, "To measure is to know." Regardless of whether measurement is qualitative or quantitative, measurement is required to scientifically understand the present state of objects and how they may be improved. Indeed, measurement of vague constructs can help to develop new ideas about them. The measurement of many entities is straightforward, e.g. the distance between 2 points or the mass of a rock. However, it is in the measurement of the intangible that formal measurement comes into considerable importance. In such cases, knowing how to measure is vital. The measurement of quality is an example of such intangible entities. For example, one can speak of quality of life, quality of service and quality of construction, but the interpretation of quality will differ from person to person because it is a subjective measure. With regards to controlled experimental quality, this issue is no different. Despite a general understanding of experimental quality (though this is not always consistent as described in Chapter 3), the problem remains. How then is it possible to transform a subjective entity into an objective measurement? The field of psychometrics deals with this quandary.

2.3. Scales and Measurement Theories

Psychometrics has provided a wealth of knowledge on how to measure that which is not directly observable. The use of psychometric techniques has allowed measurement of intelligence (IQ scores), scholastic ability, social phenomena and mental health (125). In Chapter 3, it will be seen that psychometric methods have been applied to measure quality of medical trials.

2.3.1. Theoretical Models of Experimental Quality

If measurement is important, then there should be an understanding of what is measurement. It was described by the eminent psychologist, Stanley Smith Stevens, as "the assignment of numerals to objects or events according to rules." (126) Stevens highlighted the need for explicit understanding of the rules for numerical assignment and the mathematical properties of what is being measured. Therefore, measurement is as much understanding the nature of the phenomenon being measured, as it is the actual process. Other than the physical sciences (e.g. measurement of length and weight), this is no trivial task especially in the social and behavioural sciences. Indeed, Stevens' work regarding the subjective auditory sensation of loudness was criticised because "any law purporting to express a quantitative relation between sensation intensity and stimulus intensity is not merely false but is in fact meaningless unless a meaning can be given to the concept of addition as applied to sensation." (126) This problem is encountered in the measurement of informatics experimental quality. What are the rules and mathematical properties that govern the measurement of quality? These are largely unknown as a theoretical model is mostly ignored (in Chapter 3 it will be seen that definitions of experimental quality are frequently unacknowledged.)

Stevens' ideas of measurement level can be helpful in constructing theoretical models of experimental quality, i.e. nominal, ordinal, interval and ratio (126). Nominal level assigns numerals as labels in the same way that letters could be applied. Assignment can be to individuals, e.g. the assignment of unique football jersey numbers, or of individuals of the same type to a class, e.g. a survey coding males as 0 and females as 1. The meaning of the numerals is therefore arbitrary. It is however consistent with the definition of measurement since rules are followed; the rule is numerals should be unique for individuals or classes. The only admissible transformation of nominal data is one-to-one substitution, e.g. labelling males instead as 2 (an admissible transformation is a mathematical manipulation that preserves the empirical observation (16).) The ordinal level requires that the rules for nominal scale be adhered to and that a rank order exists. Examples of ordinal measurement include placement in a competition, i.e. first, second, third, etc and severity of software failure, i.e. negligible, marginal, critical, catastrophic (16). Because rank order pays no attention to the consistency of differences between ranks, means and standard deviations are inappropriate. The admissible transformation is any monotonic increasing function (thus preserving rank order). Interval level of measurement assumes the requirements of nominal and ordinal measurement, that the distance between ranks is consistent and that a zero point is arbitrary. Temperature in Celsius and Fahrenheit are often-quoted examples. A difference of 1 degree is consistent in meaning over the temperature scales, and the zero points are by convention. Admissible transformations preserve interval equality. Lastly, ratio measurement assumes the requirements of the previous three, except that the zero point is not arbitrary, and ratios are equal. With regards to this last criterion, interval measurement does not conform to equality of ratios. Multiplication is inadmissible for interval data but not for ratio data. For instance, it is incorrect to state that a temperature of 40 degrees Celsius today is twice as hot as 20 degrees yesterday. After Fahrenheit conversion, 104 degrees is not twice that of 68 degrees. However, it is correct to state that 20cm is twice that of 10cm because ratio is preserved when converting to inches (7.8" and 3.9"). Admissible transformations therefore preserve ratio. Many attributes in physics are ratio, e.g. absolute temperature, periods of time, length and mass, as are counts, e.g. income.

How can a theoretical model of experimental quality be related to level of measurement? One suggestion (126) is that the object of measurement should satisfy a level in a top to bottom approach. First, therefore, can quality be considered at a ratio level? Is there a natural zero point? The answer is unknown, and thus ratio level of measurement does not characterise experimental quality. This would have implication for ratio description between studies, e.g. instead of stating study A had twice the quality of study B, it could only be said that A was greater than B by so much. The next level down is interval. Can it be said that the distance between ranks is consistent? Again, this is unknown. Hence experimental quality is not strictly interval in nature. The next level down is ordinal. Is there a rank order of experimental quality? The answer is yes. Intuitively, it is recognisable that some experiments are more credible than others because of their rigour and conduct. Formally, this is recognised by research organisations, such as the NHMRC and its

33

evidence levels (103). According to the top down approach (126), experimental quality is theoretically ordinal.

2.3.2. Experimental Quality as an Interval Measure

The problem with ordinal measurement is its limited usefulness. The assignment of numerals to ordinal states only represents rank. The numerals do not have further mathematical properties, i.e. only greater or less than comparisons. Indeed, numerals do not need to be used at all, e.g. Likert scales often contain "strongly disagree" to "strongly agree" labels. Furthermore, statistically there are limitations with the use of means and standard deviations and possibly statistical tests, though this remains in debate (127, 128). For the purpose of measuring experimental quality, it is more useful to assume that the difference between ranks is equal and treat scales as interval. This assumption appears controversial, but assumptions of interval (or ratio) level are made often in health care and social science research. Despite incomplete understanding of intelligence (129), interval measurement instruments, such as the Weschler Adult Intelligence Scale, are commonly used. It is assumed that a visual analog scale for pain has a constant difference (amount of pain) for a fixed length between sets of points. When clinical judges assess the appropriateness of therapeutic decision making of human and artificial intelligences, there is the assumption that skill is interval. In terms of medical experimentation quality, the many scales based on interval measurement (109) suggest that the interval assumption has been accepted. However, it cannot be known whether quality is truly interval. Instead it is more useful for researchers to apply appropriate meaning and therefore appropriate mathematical operations. Numbers do not know from where they come, as Lord communicated satirically by statistically treating football jersey numbers as other than nominal (130). It is up to those applying a measurement system to justifiably assign the meaning of jersey numbers. It is, for instance, this reason that intelligence is not ratio in nature. While it might be mathematically possible to arrive at a zero value for intelligence, this has no meaning to the researcher. The issue of meaningful interpretation is discussed further in Chapter 4. For experimental quality, it is likely to remain an unresolved topic for debate. Though, as Streiner and Norman state in regards to the problem of interval assumption applied generally, "from a pragmatic viewpoint, it appears that under most circumstances, unless the distribution of scores is severely skewed, one can analyse data from rating scales as if they were interval without introducing severe bias." (131) (p. 42)

2.3.3. Theoretical and Atheoretical Measures

As DeVellis points out (125) (p. 8), it is important to acknowledge the difference between theoretical and atheoretical measures and what is being achieved in measurement. Atheoretical measurement captures descriptive data for which there is little or no theoretical foundation (the interest is in the response itself), e.g. a questionnaire that inquires about a software engineer's favourite programming language (a vendor might want to conduct a survey to assess how they should promote their latest Integrated Development Environment.) However, a measurement instrument may explore relationships and thus establish theoretical foundations, e.g. favoured programming language as a proxy for skill in maintaining object-oriented code. The construct of experimental quality has a theoretical foundation, but it can also be measured atheoretically. This book's research is concerned with theoretical measurement and the theoretical foundations of experiment quality. A related theoretical issue is why develop instruments to measure experimental quality. To some, the identification of a good experiment is perhaps as obvious as the identification of age or gender (concrete and accessible phenomena (125) that do not require complex instruments to measure). The belief of this research is that experimental quality in informatics is complex, abstract and inaccessible, like ethnicity (125). Indeed, the large number of elicited and not always agreeing experimental concepts discussed in Chapter 3 is testimony.

2.3.4. What is a Scale?

To measure intangible entities, the tool often used is the scale. Scales are instruments that purport to measure constructs not easily observable and usually take the form of a written questionnaire, form or test. To be useful, scales must demonstrate reliability and validity, which are discussed below, and are therefore said to have good psychometric properties. Scales contain items, which are the units that record an observation. Often these are questions (the item stem) with a set of responses, which may be continuous or categorical. The set of responses is sometimes itself referred to as a scale, e.g. "measured on a scale of 1 to 10". The end result of a scale instrument is usually a number quantifying the construct under study. How might scales be of use to measure the quality of controlled experiments in informatics? They may help:

- Investigators designing an experiment to avoid pitfalls or acknowledge trade-offs (a check list essentially).

- Readers of experimental reports trying to understand whether the results are credible/useful, e.g. practitioners seeking evidence and the research community.

- Journal and conference reviewers trying to assess whether a report is good enough for publication (this addresses Tichy's concern that computer science reviewers themselves may not have adequate experience (102).)

- Meta-analysts trying to weight the results of an experiment according to its quality.

- Quality improvement by providing a tool for quality monitoring.

2.3.5. Scales vs. Indexes

The measurement questionnaire of this research, the MICE index, is strictly not a scale (the term scale is often used loosely in general to mean any psychometrically developed measurement instrument.) The difference between scales and indexes is the former is related to effect while the latter is related to cause. Scales (should) contain homogenous items. Each item "taps different aspects of the same attribute." (131) (p. 68) Therefore, items should be related to each other. In other words, the observations recorded by each item are the effect of the attribute/construct (the items share a common cause (125) (p. 11).) An anxiety scale might have items inquiring about sweatiness, worry and irritability (131) (p. 74). A scale measuring employee laziness might include items such as time to complete tasks, absenteeism and work errors (132). The opposite is true for indexes. Indexes are not homogeneous. Each item determines the attribute rather than being the effect of the attribute (the items share a common consequence (125) (p. 11). The Australian Consumer Price Index (CPI) is comprised of 11 major household expenditures that are not necessarily related to each other, e.g. food, health, education, transportation (133). Each item determines (causes) the CPI (the CPI is built up of the items.) An index that measures programmer skill might include items such as duration of work experience, grades at university and number of large projects completed.

The recognition of indexes and scales is not merely academic. Measures of consistency such as Cronbach's alpha can be applied to scales but not to indexes. Other psychometric techniques that assume homogeneity also cannot be applied, e.g. factor analysis (131) (p. 75). Also the effect of individual items is more important to indexes than scales. Because scale items (ideally) correlate with each other, the absence of one item may not affect the final score from a scale. However, the absence of an item in an index may dramatically affect the final score because it is possible that no other items tap similar aspects. Unfortunately, the difference between scales and indexes can be seen as a continuum, and there are examples of questionnaires that have properties of both (134). Part of the problem is a lack of understanding of the theory behind the constructs being measured (for a more in depth discussion, see (134).)

2.3.6. Scales, Indexes and Experimental Quality

The concept of scales versus indexes has implication in developing questionnaires for experimental quality. The issue of whether experimental quality should be measured by scale or index is not explicitly mentioned in the literature described in Chapter 3. The preceding discussion shows that application of psychometric techniques depends on an understanding of how experimental quality (the construct) relates to items. For instance, the article by de Keizer and Ammenwerth (135) describes the authors' instrument to measure the quality of health informatics evaluation reports. Their instrument contains items, which are scored and summed as a final total indicating the quality of the evaluation. However, it is difficult to see how the item on introduction clarity and relevant referencing is correlated with appropriate methods of data analysis or the item about discussion and generalisability of results. In other words, the instrument is not unidimensional. The instrument would constitute an index, yet the authors mention testing internal consistency (correlation among the items). MICE, on the other hand, is explicitly an index since the items determine the quality score and are not necessarily inter-related, e.g. the item inquiring about confidence intervals is not related to the one inquiring about clarity of experimental rationale. Generally speaking, the importance of items to indexes can be considered in terms of the length of indexes and therefore comprehensiveness validity (see below for a description of validity.) A short index is likely to be affected by the absence of important items since there may be few related items. Some might consider the MICE index a long questionnaire, but its psychometric properties are improved as a result. The issue of brevity of scales is discussed later.

2.3.7. Classical Test Theories

Much psychometric measurement in the last century has been focussed on classical test theories (CTT) (136). One of the useful axioms of CTT is that observed measurement (X) consists of a true component (T) and an error component (E) (125, 131, 136-138), i.e.

$$X = T + E$$

The MICE index observes the component X, but the true value of experimental quality is clouded by noise E. The true component T is the actual quality of an experiment and is what instruments attempt to measure. Therefore, measurement should seek to understand how much error is present. The equation forms the foundation of reliability but is not very useful in this form because E is unknown. Instead, estimates of error can be achieved through repeated measurement of the same construct and assessing inter-item correlations (for unidimensional constructs) or test-retest properties (137, 139).

CTT is described here since it has importance for the reliability assessment of the MICE index. There are other measurement theories, which are potentially useful in research such as this. Generalisability theory (140) is an extension of CTT and allows for more complex modelling of measurement and, in particular, for multiple sources of error and determination of their extents, i.e. generalisation of a scale's properties to a wider set of situations (139) (e.g. not just focussing on the particular instance of when a test is taken). CTT assumes that there is only one source of error as represented by the E term. CTT for example cannot distinguish between the error associated with internal consistency of items and error associated with application of the same scale on different occasions (test-retest) (139). However, because of its technical simplicity, CTT has been more widely adopted (139).

2.4. General Steps in Scale Development

This section does not attempt to be a comprehensive guide to scale or index development but provides an established framework upon which the MICE index was created. While there is no single recipe for developing scales, general steps exist.

2.4.1. What is the Construct?

The first step, according to DeVellis (125), is understanding the attribute being measured. This is not trivial. Scales come into use because they tap intangible attributes. The discussion above about level of measurement of experimental quality illustrates non-triviality. Attributes are often based in theory. What theories exist about controlled experimental quality in informatics? Informatics has borrowed ideas from medical and psychological experimentation. Health informatics experimental theory is strongly derived from clinical trial theory. A definition of the attribute is most useful (this includes making explicit its breadth or scope.) A definition of experimental quality is provided in Chapter 3. Is the attribute to be measured by an index or a scale? Is the attribute meaningfully measurable by (or in) the group who will use the instrument or will different groups affect responses? DeVellis (125) (p. 63) provides the illustrative example of an item that inquires about a person's ability to "get going" and how this can be influenced by whether such an item is answered by a depressed individual or an arthritic one. What level of capability is assumed for a scale user to actually complete the scale meaningfully? Thus, a scale should have a defined user group.

2.4.2. Item Pool

The second step (125) is to generate an item pool. Because instrument development is time consuming, effort should be directed at seeing whether existing scales or scale items are adequate, i.e. already proven to be rigorous and useful. A new scale is justified when no other instruments exist, if other scales are deficient or if a new scale is cheaper or easier to apply (131) (p. 8). Deficiencies can include poorly defined constructs, poor reliability and untested validity. Previous scales can still be reused even if they are not overall adequately reliable or valid, since individual items may be sound. Hence reviewing previous scales can help reduce the amount of work for item generation. In Chapter 3, it will be seen that instruments to measure experimental quality in informatics demonstrate these deficiencies and give justification for the MICE index. Initially, an

38

item pool should be highly inclusive. This helps comprehensiveness validity, which is explained below. Having many items initially also improves the reliability of a scale. This can be demonstrated by the Spearman-Brown prophecy formula (131) (p. 71):

$$r_{sb} = \frac{kr}{1+(k-1)r}$$

where r_{sb} is the predicted reliability given the current reliability (r) and the factor by which the items are increased or decreased (k). Figure 1 illustrates, for a scale with an original reliability coefficient of 0.5, the effect of reducing and adding items on subsequent reliability.

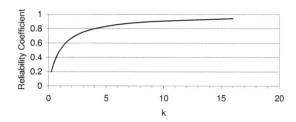

Figure 1. Effect of number of items on reliability as predicted by the Spearman-Brown formula. k is the factor by which the number of items is multiplied (< 1 is a reduction in items.)

In writing new items, attention should be paid to general comprehension (125). This includes clarity without unnecessary wordiness, appropriate reading level and avoidance of multiple negatives, double-barrelled items, negative wording and other ambiguities of written English. Such problems are especially found in questionnaire instruments aimed at lay people but can also affect questionnaires to be completed by domain specialists. Reading level refers to the number of words and syllables of sentences. Long complex sentences are more difficult to understand, although may be necessary to explain what an item is seeking. Multiple negatives refers to the use of more than one negative expression, e.g. "I do not believe the rationale is unclear," is harder to understand than, "I believe the rationale is clear." Double-barrelled items convey more than one idea, e.g. "The introduction, method, results and discussion are well-written." What if only one is well-written? This may be acceptable if all elements are required to be good. Negatively worded items attempt to capture the absence of something rather than its presence (positive wording), e.g. "The statistical methods are inappropriate," versus, "The statistical methods are appropriate." This issue is not as much of a problem with the MICE index as with lay-public questionnaires. The benefit of making some items negative is to prevent responders from answering "yes" to everything because of poor cognition or motivation (131). This is less likely to affect the MICE index because users will be well-educated and motivated (they would not be using the index otherwise.) Generally, however, negative wording should be avoided since it is cognitively more demanding. Also, simply inversing the polarity does not always inverse meaning, e.g. answering "no" to "I feel unwell" is not semantically the same as answering "yes" to "I feel well" (131) (p. 64).

2.4.3. Item Format

The next step in scale development is consideration of the general format (125). The format of scales can be classified according to items' levels of measurement: categorical (nominal) and continuous (ordinal, interval, ratio) (131). Some scales are purely categorical and some are purely continuous, but often scales utilise both types of items. When considering the general format, attention should be paid to whether items best fall into categorical or continuous measurement. Categorical items only allow nominal responses such as "yes/no", "true/false" or placing a check mark. Many attributes lie on a continuum; therefore, a completely categorical format should be used with caution. The Jadad scale is an example of a completely categorical scale (141). According to Norman and Streiner, problems from categorical questions can arise. Firstly, providing only 2 extremes of response can cause confusion to users when they wish to respond along a continuum, e.g. for Jadad's item, "Was there a description of withdrawals and dropouts?", scale users may be confused whether a minor (and inadequate) description still counts as a description. In contrast, Chalmer's (142) item provided alternative responses about how withdrawals were handled. The second problem relates to reduction in the reliability coefficient of a scale when continuous variables are dichotomised (131) (p. 32). However, for some questions, categorical responses are appropriate, i.e. when scale users would find it difficult to make finer discriminations that binary ones (the added cognitive burden can introduce error.) Another issue raised with categorical responses is how to score them (more precisely, how to treat categorical responses as continuous). This is discussed in Chapter 4.

Continuous formats include direct estimation and comparative methods (131) (p. 32). The direct estimation methods require the user to directly indicate their quantitative response on a continuum. The response may be visually quantifiable, such as using a line upon which users indicate their answer (pain is often quantified using these so-called visual analog scales.) The response may be a series of adjectives along a continuum, which may be unipolar or bipolar. Unipolar responses increase from none or a small amount, e.g. "never", "rarely", "sometimes", "often", "always". Bipolar scales (Likert scales are a type) have negative, middle and positive levels of adjectives, e.g. "strongly disagree", "disagree", "neutral", "agree", "strongly agree". The Goodman scale is an example of mostly adjectival bipolar continuous responses (143). With comparative methods, the value of an item is determined by how the item ranks in comparison to other items. That is, the value is not directly obtained from the user. Various techniques are used to rank items. Thurstone's equal-appearing intervals method uses a group of judges (not the actual scale users) to rank (pre-calibrate) items. Scale users then agree or disagree with items, and the final scale score is computed based on the rank of each item (as determined by the judging step). Guttman scaling ranks each item into successively higher levels of the attribute. An endorsed item implicitly means that lower items are also endorsed. In pre-testing, item values are determined by how well items are ranked against each other. Scale users are asked to agree or disagree with items. Both types of formats assume unidimensional attributes. Comparative methods are used in social and health scales, but they cannot be easily applied to experimental quality assessment, especially if quality is not unidimensional. Neither format is used in the scales examined in this research. That is, all the experimental quality scales discovered in the literature by this research have used categorical, direct estimation or mixed (both) formats.

Continuous items require further consideration (131). One of the main issues in designing continuous items is deciding how many response steps should be made available to scale users. Many of the scales discovered in this reserach use 3 steps (in the style of complete, partial and none) while the Goodman scale uses mainly 5. In general measurement, scales often utilise 5 to 7 steps. Miller's seminal work demonstrated that a person's ability to discriminate often falls between 5 and 9 categories (144). Hence using 5 to 9 steps has become a de facto standard in scale development. Another common issue is the scale user's interpretation of adjectival responses. Words such as "almost always", "often", "seldom" and "rarely" demonstrate a wide variance in meaning (131) (p. 40). There is general human variation in the interpretation of language. Additionally descriptors can carry different meaning depending on the context of a scale and how the scale user is placed in that context. In the context of scale users who are assessing the quality of controlled experiments, there is variance associated with educational background of users. For example, the degree to which a user is familiar with experimental methods will influence the interpretation of adjectives such as "suitable", "moderately suitable" and "unsuitable" when applied to experimental design. Where possible, objective numerical responses should be used. Though, if this were the case for an entire scale, the scale would probably not be necessary; it is in the measurement of the subjective that scales come into power. If adjectival continuous responses are used, error will be introduced and should be measured as part of reliability testing. A third issue in continuous (and categorical) response creation is whether numbers should be placed under each step (or category). Schwarz et al (145) found that scale users are likely to be influenced by numbers placed with response steps or categories. Participants were randomly allocated to complete an 11-

point scale for measuring personal success in life, with the only difference being the numerals applied (0 to 10 or −5 to 5) to response adjectives ("not successful at all" to "extremely successful"). 34% of users answered in the first half of the scale compared to 13% (second group), suggesting the negative integers dissuaded users. It is theorised that numerals assist in disambiguating response labels. The MICE index uses mainly 7 response steps with adjectival and numerical labels.

The order of questions should also be planned. How questions are answered is influenced by previous questions because scale users want to appear consistent and also subsequent questions may prompt a scale user's memory leading to modification of earlier questions (131) (p . 41). This has implication for experimental quality scales since experiments usually follow a set path (planning, conduct, analysis and reporting), and reports often follow a set format (introduction, method, results, discussion). Questions should follow similar progressions. For example, an item relating to adequacy of discussion should not come before one on bias, as the latter may prompt a change in the former.

2.4.4.   Item Review

The next step in scale development is review of the initial item pool by experts (125). The goals of this activity are to check that each item is relevant to the construct and is clear in understanding and to raise further items that have been omitted. Experts are those who are knowledgeable in the content that the scale measures. In the case of experimental quality, these might be statisticians and academic empirical researchers. The decision to accept or reject their advice is ultimately left to the scale developer (125), and items are modified accordingly (this is especially important if content experts are not be familiar with scale development principles.)

2.4.5.   Score Weights

The scoring system for the scale should be defined as part of item creation. Each item's response steps or categories are assigned a value, and these values are often summed to produce a final score. The scale developer must decide how to use each value in the final score. Developers can define each item to have equal contribution to a final score (a weighting of 1 for each item). If some items are thought to be more important than others in tapping a construct, then higher weights are applied to those items. Randomised allocation of treatment in controlled experiments is often considered to be an important determinant of quality and is often weighted heavily in scales, e.g. the Balas (146) and Chalmers (142) scales. While it makes intuitive sense that important items should contribute more heavily to a scale score, there are 2 problems. The first is that the weight is (usually) arbitrarily assigned rather than based on empirical evidence, e.g. how is it known that randomisation is 10 times more important in experimental quality than appropriate statistical analysis? The second is that, for long scales, computation of the score becomes burdensome. Streiner and Norman suggest that for long enough scales (perhaps more than 20 to 40 items) weighting does not significantly affect the rank order of scores. They point to empirical evidence showing that long scales remain consistent in rank ordering of objects when various weighting schemes are used (131) (p. 103-104). They suggest that, "differential weighting contributes relatively little, except added complexity for the scorer." (131) (p. 104) This means the best approach to scoring may be to simply sum the item responses, providing the scale contains 40 or so items. For this reason and for comprehensiveness validity, the MICE index contains sufficient items.

2.4.6. Scale Testing and Refinement

At this point, a draft set of items should be ready for testing. Testing involves applying the questionnaire to a sample and assessing the items for reliability and validity, which are discussed below. The sample that is chosen should be representative of that which the scale will finally measure. In psychometric scales that assess human attributes, this involves sampling people to complete questionnaires. With experimental quality scales, this involves choosing a sample of experiments for assessment. The size of a sample in human psychometric testing was recommended by Nunnally to be 300 participants (147) and at least 100 by Friedman and Wyatt (138) (p. 126). More accurately, the number of objects on which to test a scale is that which will provide high reliability and be representative of a population. Larger samples will reduce variability and be more representative. Since reliability is also related to the number of items and to the number of observations made on objects, sample sizes can be smaller than what might be prescribed. For representativeness, it is much more difficult to know and assess whether a sample is adequate. In terms of quantitative experimental quality, a representative sample might show a wide range of scores (reflecting the range seen in the population), which might be normally distributed. If it is known from previous evidence how experimental quality scores behave, then a similarly behaving sample could be said to be representative. Unfortunately, this is largely unknown for informatics experiments. There are also practical limitations on sample sizes, e.g. the population from which to choose may be small or limited time and resources that a researcher has to draw large samples. The MICE index used a sample size of 58 experimental informatics studies, and reliability was high, but representativeness is more difficult to gauge.

When the scale has been applied to a sample of objects, its reliability can be statistically analysed. The scale should then be tested formally for its validity. These are discussed in the following sections. Once shown to be reliable and valid, the length of the scale should be shortened without

43

sacrificing the aforementioned properties and gains associated with longer scales. Because CTT assumes that error is randomly distributed with a mean of 0 (125, 136), the inclusion of more items increases the likelihood of error cancelling each other out for an individual item. On the other hand, scales that are too long are mentally taxing and can suffer degraded performance. The Spearman-Brown prophecy formula can give guidance on the effect of reducing the number of items on reliability, but the removal of items may also change the interpretation of items and the scale. Hence, measures of reliability and validity should be recalculated. Various methods can be used to shorten a scale. Items that have poor individual reliability over repeated measurement can be removed. Items responses that are frequently endorsed (all or most scales users answer an item with the same response) do not discriminate well between objects and can be removed. The threshold is arbitrary, e.g. 95% of scale users selecting the same response. Chapter 3 discusses the methods used to shorten the MICE index from 80 to 38 items.

When a reliable and valid instrument is produced and made more efficient, it can be used for the purposes for which it was designed. However, development does not necessarily end there. Usage by other researchers can stimulate further work to fine-tune instruments; the ongoing revising of scales in sociology and psychology is testament to this.

2.5.   Reliability

Consistency of measurement is fundamental to scale development. If a scale cannot produce a similar (or ideally the same) result when measuring the same object under the same conditions, the difference must be due to error under the assumptions of CTT and positivistic philosophy. Like a ruler suffering from parallax error, if a scale is highly erroneous, it is of little use.

Reliability theory is based on CTT as discussed earlier in this chapter. A useful form of reliability is the variance (variability) of an object in relation to total variance, since the error component E cannot be directly known. By repeating measurements of the same objects, variance can be known, and reliability can be expressed in the form of an intraclass correlation coefficient (ICC):

$$\rho = \frac{\sigma^2_{objects}}{\sigma^2_{objects} + \sigma^2_{raters} + \sigma^2_{error}}$$

where ρ is reliability, σ^2 is variance, and the denominator is the total variance. In the case of experimental quality, the studies are objects (in psychometric research of people, the objects would be people.) Raters are judges who perform the measurement.

Measurement of studies by judges produces a matrix of observations against objects (138) (p. 122) as shown in Table 1 and Table 6 (Chapter 3). Observations can be made by different judges (inter-rater reliability) or by single judge at different periods in time (test-retest reliability).

Objects	Observations				
	Rater 1	Rater 2	Rater 3	Rater 4	Mean
A	Score A1	Score A2	Score A3	Score A4	A
B	Score B1	Score B2	Score B3	Score B4	B
C	Score C1	Score C2	Score C3	Score C4	C
D	Score D1	Score D2	Score D3	Score D4	D
Mean	R1	R2	R3	R4	

Table 1. Sample objects-by-observations matrix.

From such table data, mean squares can be calculated and used in an analysis of variance (ANOVA) table. The output of ANOVA will be variances of studies and error. These can be entered into the reliability formula above (alternatively, a mean squares formula can be used instead of variance.) For further details on mean squares and ANOVA, the reader is advised to consult textbooks on statistical analysis. The ICC formula presented above is only one form of the ICC. Further details can be found in Shrout and Fleiss' seminal paper on the subject (148). However, there are 2 aspects of the ICC that require discussion. Firstly experimental quality scores should be consistent with respect to their absolute agreement (whether numerical value is consistent over repeated measurement rather than just consistent rank order). This is important if the scores will be used against an external criterion, e.g. a cut-off for deciding what is acceptable experimental quality. Secondly, the ICC used in this research is a two-way model since the author evaluated all studies.

The above description of intraclass correlation coefficients is one method of calculating reliability coefficients. Another method is the kappa coefficient for agreement between judges for dichotomous objects. Another major form of reliability is internal consistency, usually measured with Cronbach's alpha (149). Internal consistency reliability refers to whether items are correlated with each other and only applies to homogeneous scales. It cannot be applied to the MICE index. The appropriate choice of reliability measure is often a matter of debate (131) (p. 138). It depends on the properties of the construct and the resources (time, judges) available to generate reliability data. Inter-rater reliability can be usefully applied to the assessment of experimental studies but requires considerable effort on the part of a few judges to review many experimental reports (or alternatively many judges to review fewer reports) in order to achieve stable estimates of reliability. Depending on research resources, this may not be feasible. On the other hand, test-retest reliability can be less resource intense but raises the issue of different interpretation of items by different judges. Also, memory effects can be a concern (where judges remember previous assessment and simply reiterate rather than performing de novo evaluation). Providing a construct is stable over time, test-retest can be a rigorous form of reliability (125) (p. 44), (131) (p. 144). The advantages and disadvantages of using test-retest reliability for this work are explored in Chapter 6.

2.6.   Validity

The validity of an instrument refers to whether it measures that which it purports to measure. In the physical sciences, validity is often straightforward, e.g. height, weight, temperature, velocity are readily observable, and the instruments that measure them do not need to undergo formal validity testing. To be more accurate, the theories of the constructs are well-understood. For example, the construct of height is well-understood. For this reason, a tape measure does not need validation. It is not the instrument that is important but rather the construct. In contrast, many psychological, social and medical constructs are not readily observable and are not fully understood in theory. Instruments that measure intelligence, skill, attitudes and many clinical syndromes thus require validation. Similarly, quality of controlled experiments is a construct whose theoretical foundation is more complicated than, say, temperature. Therefore, quality scales should be formally tested with respect to validity.

2.6.1.   Validity as Hypothesis Testing

Traditionally, validity has been categorised into face, content, criterion and construct types. Streiner and Norman provide a different view of validity that highlights the importance of formal assessment (131) (p. 174). Validity is said to be a process of hypothesis testing that allows inferences to be made about the objects scored by a scale. With a valid scale, one can make more confident inferences about the object, e.g. if the scale assesses a study to be of poor quality then in all other aspects of quality the study is indeed poor, or if a scale assesses a person to have low intelligence then in other tests of intelligence the person would likely do badly. Therefore, validity becomes a matter of testing whether hypotheses about scales and constructs are supported. The implications for validity testing are that one test is insufficient and that, "scale constructors are limited only by their imagination in devising experiments to test their hypotheses." (131) (p. 174) Several hypotheses are required to produce enough evidence of validity and to triangulate aspects of intangible constructs. Furthermore, when a construct is not understood well, any hypothesis test may provide useful information. These points become particularly clear when thinking about what construct validity tests to apply to experimental quality. This research uses several methods of validation and hypothesis testing. As discussed in Chapter 6, not all hypotheses were ideal, and there is room for further research.

46

2.6.2. Face Validity

Face validity refers to whether, on face value, the instrument measures what it is trying to measure. This is the least stringent of the validity types and is usually all that is required for well-understood constructs, e.g. rulers, on face value, measure length and not weight. Face value has some potential limitations. While a high consensus would be achieved for saying a ruler measures length, a scale measuring experimental quality might be interpreted by some as a measure of report quality (e.g. conciseness, grammar, use of tables etc) or the experiment itself (e.g. appropriate design, control for bias, use of statistical methods etc). Therefore, face value requires some consensus on the theory of a construct. For experimental quality in informatics (and even in medicine), there remains variability between researchers as will be seen in Chapter 3. Related to this is the problem of the scale developers' perspective. If a research group assesses their scale on face value, they are likely to be satisfied because their view of experimental quality will be incorporated into the instrument. Also, face value is often assumed rather than empirically shown unlike the stringent criterion and construct validities discussed below. Face validity is a necessary step, but it is not sufficient to determine validity. Unfortunately for experimental quality scales in health informatics, researchers have not taken their instruments past presumably face validity (112, 135, 146, 150). The disadvantage of more stringent forms is that they require further research effort.

2.6.3. Content/Comprehensiveness Validity

Content validity reflects the extent to which a scale captures the breadth of the construct and is therefore also called comprehensiveness validity. However, it has been described as synonymous with face validity (138) (p. 131). In this work, the former definition is used. If a scale is content valid, it will allow greater inferring about the objects it measures (131) (p. 175). For example, someone who does well on an exam that tests a large number of concepts can be inferred with greater confidence to have superior knowledge over a poorer examinee, than if the exam consists of only 1 question. A risk, therefore, with short scales, is that the inferences that can be made may be severely limited. This point is even more important for heterogeneous constructs. The breadth of a construct may be well-defined, e.g. the range of physical examination skills required of a medical student to perform at an Objective Structured Clinical Examination (151), but more often constructs are broad. Experimental quality is a broad construct that, as will be seen in Chapter 3, can be conceptualised in hundreds of ideas and "practice tips". As such, scales measuring experimental quality should probably also be appropriately lengthy in order to be comprehensive.

2.6.4. Criterion Validity

Criterion and construct validity are stronger forms of validity because they are amenable to formal comparison and hypothesis testing. Criterion validity refers to whether a scale correlates well with an external "gold" standard. If an object scores highly on the scale, will it also score highly on the gold standard? For continuous data, a series of objects can be assessed by both instruments and plotted on a graph with each axis representing a scale. Simple correlation can be measured, e.g. Pearson product moment correlation. When both instruments are applied to objects at the same time, concurrent (criterion) validity testing is being employed. When the result by which the prototype scale will be compared can only be known in the future, predictive (criterion) validity is being used. An example of the latter is the use of university aptitude tests to predict whether a person will successfully graduate in years to come (graduation is the gold standard, which occurs in the future.) Depending on the future criterion standard, concurrent validity may be more useful in research where there is a constraint of time. Another important aspect is the determination of the gold standard. Criterion validity is useful if a reliable and valid gold standard exists. Apart from the issue of why another scale is needed if a gold standard already exists, the main problem with criterion validity is when a gold standard does not exist. In Chapter 3, it will be seen that no gold standards for measuring controlled experimental quality in informatics exist and that more research needs to be done, e.g. the use of other standards such as Journal Impact Factor (The Thompson Corporation, Stamford, USA).

2.6.5. Construct Validity

Construct validity has been traditionally viewed as whether the scale behaves in the same fashion as that expected of the construct. In this sense, construct validity is classically related to hypothesis testing. Indeed, constructs are also referred to as "hypothetical constructs" when speaking of construct validity. A scale can be tested against the hypothetical nature of the construct. If people of higher intelligence are more likely to earn a higher income, then a hypothetical test of an intelligence scale is that people of high income should have greater scores than those of low income. Despite being a strong form of validity testing (138) (p. 132), construct validity can suffer from the perplexing problem of testing construct theory and scale property at the same time (131) (p. 181). If construct validity is poor, is it because the theory of the construct is wrong, the instrument is bad or both? Because constructs are usually intangible to begin with (this is precisely why they are measured using scale theory), then separating poor construct theory from poor instrument may not be easy. It is for this reason that researchers should consider many hypotheses about their constructs, especially when theoretical foundations are not fully elucidated. As Streiner and Norman state, "There is no one single experiment which can unequivocally prove a construct. Construct validation is an on-going process, of learning more about the construct, making new predictions, and then testing them." (131) (p. 180) Because it is not well-understood how experimental quality should behave, several hypotheses are needed.

Construct validity has also been divided into subtypes: convergent and divergent. When a construct is hypothesised to highly correlate with related variables, it is said to demonstrate convergent validity. When the hypothesis is that of low or no correlation with unrelated variables, this is known as divergent validity. Both are useful forms as they approach the understanding of constructs from opposite ends and provide further triangulation.

2.6.6. Criterion vs. Construct Validity

The distinction between criterion and construct validity can be blurred, and this supports Streiner and Norman's interpretation of validity as simply hypothesis testing. Indeed, criterion validity can be thought of as testing the following hypothesis: people or objects that do well on one scale should also do well on another that taps the same attribute. DeVellis goes on about the confusion, stating that the same statistical correlation test can be used for both construct and criterion validity (125) (p. 53). If a difference between criterion and construct validity must be made, then it is perhaps one of intent, according to DeVellis. Construct validity correlations intend to provide evidence for explaining theoretical foundation. Criterion validity correlations do not. For instance, it might be observed that a scale measuring the complexity of a graphical user interface correlates with a learner's time to complete a task. Theory informs that humans perform less well when confronted by complexity. Thus, one would hypothesise, based on our knowledge of human cognition, that the scale should correlate with different levels of complexity. This would be a test for construct validity. On the other hand, the scale could be tested for its ability to predict a person's task completion time without the understanding of why (i.e. cognitive limits). All that needs to be shown is that interfaces that are deemed simple by the scale are associated with short times, and complex interfaces with long times, and that this was the same finding using a gold standard. This would be a test for criterion validity. Yet, the battery of tests could be the same; in both cases, the scale is applied to a set of simple and complex interfaces (complexity determined by something or someone else), and the performance times are measured. The method and results could be the same, but one approach is based on theoretical ideas of how complexity and cognition behave and how the scale should subsequently behave; the other does not. It is a subtle distinction. This issue is raised here because the known-groups method used in Chapter 3 can be thought of as a form of either criterion or construct validity. However, the distinction does not need to be overemphasised.

Despite the overlap between criterion and construct validity and the overarching view that all validity is basically hypothesis testing, the different types of validity still largely feature in the literature and are likely to do so for some time. Therefore, this work adheres to the terminology but recognises the differences of interpretation.

2.7. Discussion

From this chapter it can be seen that there is considerable theory behind the development and testing of scales and indexes. This chapter is not meant to be a comprehensive review of psychometric scale theory but to highlight areas of background knowledge required for interpretation of the methods used and results produced for this research. The reader is encouraged to view seminal works for further instruction, e.g. Nunnally's "Psychometric Theory" (147). Instruments that attempt to measure empirical research quality must consider psychometric theory. In support of the research hypotheses, this research had to apply measurement and scale theories established in other domains. Unfortunately, Chapter 3 will show that this has not sufficiently been the case for health informatics scores. In computer science experimentation, instruments have yet to be developed; eventually they too must consider the theories presented here.

This chapter also raises a related and broader issue in informatics. Formal scale development is important for researchers measuring intangible constructs in informatics. This issue occurs commonly in health informatics and computer science research but is probably under-recognised. When measuring vague attributes, such as user satisfaction with a computer programme, researchers should be aware that this is a measurement problem. A formal approach to measurement is required and this is why psychometric theory exists. How often do informatics researchers realise the need for formal measurement and how often are proven scales re-used?

There are many paths for the informatics scale developer to take, and few in informatics are suitably educated. Moreover, there is debate among psychometricians and mathematicians on correct use of methods within the field of measurement itself. Therefore, there is likely to be disagreement on the methods used in informatics and in this research. This should not discourage adoption of formal theory, lest the alternative is unscientific measurement.

Chapter 3: Development of the MICE Index

3.1.   Overview of Development

The first hypothesis of this research was to develop a useful instrument for measuring the quality of human-based experiments in informatics. The second and third hypotheses were to develop such a tool for use within computer science and health informatics. This chapter describes the development and testing processes adopted to demonstrate the 3 hypotheses and represents the main work of this research.

The MICE index was developed following psychometric theories and the general steps of scale creation described in the previous chapter. The development stages were literature search, item generation, reliability testing, validity testing and item reduction. After questionnaire items were reduced, the reliability and validity tests were repeated, and the MICE index was deemed suitable and ready for application. The overall process is represented in Figure 2.

The literature search, from the fields of computer science, health informatics and medicine, informed what previous scales existed, what experimental concepts are considered important to quality and the definition of purpose and scope of the index. This body of knowledge of experimental quality and quality improvement was the basis for understanding the construct and generating an item pool. The items were written following principles described in Chapter 2 and underwent expert review. This produced an 80-item questionnaire (MICE-80). The MICE-80 version was tested for reliability using the test-retest method and formally tested for validity using criterion and construct validity methods. Parametric and nonparametric inference tests and correlational tests were applied to validity tests. When reliability and validity were demonstrated, the items were reduced to 38 according to a set of criteria, and the reliability and validity tests were repeated. This produced the preferred MICE index (MICE-38).

3.2.   Literature Review

The first purpose of the literature review was examine what scales existed for measuring the quality of controlled experiments in informatics. As discussed in Chapter 2, one should seek whether adequate instruments exist and whether they should be improved.

The second purpose of the review was to determine what issues and concepts in controlled experimentation are considered important or that are frequently performed inadequately. The term

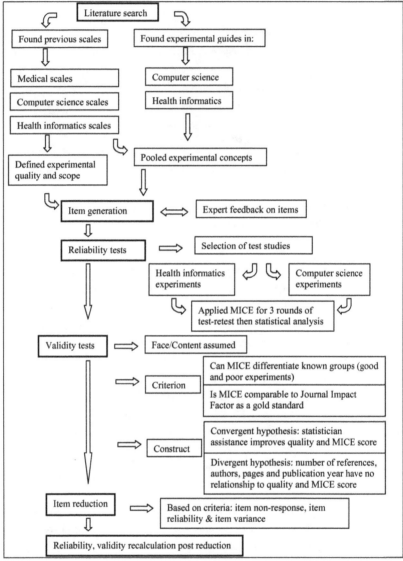

Figure 2. Overview of the development and testing of the MICE index.
Heavily outlined boxes are described in further detail in this chapter.

concept is used broadly in this book to mean principles, practice tips and pitfalls in the conduct and reporting of controlled experiments.

The third purpose was to assist in defining the purpose and scope of the new scale. Related to this was the need to define as much as possible what is meant by experimental quality.

3.2.1. Search Strategy

There were 2 arms to the literature search strategy. The left arm, as indicated in Figure 2, looked for scales from the health informatics, computer science and medical literature. The right arm looked for guidelines on experimental conduct in the health informatics and computer science literature. Both arms contributed to the generation of important experimental concepts. The search for scales was focussed on the computer science and health informatics literature since a scale's scope must be appropriate to the setting. While there are many medical scales for measuring clinical trial quality, they cannot be applied to health informatics and, indeed, informatics in general because a scale's scope and setting must be predefined. The rationale for examining some scales from clinical trial literature was to provide examples of scale development on which to base an informatics scale. Similarly, while there is wealth of literature on experimental conduct from a variety of disciplines, e.g. sociology, medicine and mathematics, the purpose of examining experimental guidelines from informatics was to understand how the setting of informatics affects the conduct of experiments. Hence it was appropriate to examine the experimental literature from informatics. However, there was, of course, some overlap of issues common to all experimental disciplines.

With regards to the computer science literature, the ACM Digital Library (ACM, New York, USA) and IEEE Xplore (IEEE, New York, USA) bibliographic databases were searched with the following search term strategies: "controlled experiment" AND "guideline", "controlled experiment" AND "score", "controlled experiment" AND "scale", "controlled experiment" AND "quality", "controlled experiment" AND "framework", "experiment" AND "guideline", "experiment" AND "score", "experiment" AND "scale", "experiment" AND "quality", "experiment" AND "framework". Where more than 200 matches were returned, the first 200 most relevant articles (according to the search engines) were selected for examination. In addition, the online search function of the journal Empirical Software Engineering was searched with the terms "controlled experiment", "experiment", "guideline", "scale" and "score" (individual terms).

It is noteworthy that the term "controlled experiment" is not used consistently as a keyword in the ACM Digital Library and IEEE Xplore databases. Far fewer matches were returned when using "controlled experiment" versus "experiment". Since "experiment" can be used to define a variety of experimental studies, it was expected that many of matches would not be relevant to controlled experimentation. However, reading through returned articles revealed that some were indeed reports of controlled experiments but not retrieved using "controlled experiment". This issue of inconsistent terminology when reporting controlled experiments has been noted in the computer science literature (113).

With regards to the health informatics literature, publication sources were selected by 2 methods: health informatics journals listed in ISI Web of Knowledge Journal Citation Reports (The Thompson Corporation, Stamford, USA); journals/conferences listed in PubMed (The US National Library of Medicine, Bethesda, USA) retrieved by using the Search Journals function and entering the keywords of "health informatics" and "medical informatics". Publication sources were then searched using the journal's online search interfaces and/or with PubMed's search function. The following terms were used: "trial", "experiment", "scale", "score", "guideline". Table 2 shows the list of health informatics publication sources.

The PubMed database was also used to retrieve clinical trial quality scales but in a less rigorous manner than the computing and health informatics searches. This was intended to provide examples of controlled experiment quality scales, rather than to have been an exhaustive search. The main source of clinical trial scales was the frequently cited review by Moher et al, which examined 25 such scales (109). These scales were classified as "generic" and "specific". The generic scales were applicable to all settings of clinical trials and were thus used as examples for the MICE index. 11 of the 13 published, generic scales were retrieved as full-text manuscripts. One was not in English; one was unobtainable. The well-known CONSORT guidelines and another paper from the PubMed search were also chosen.

The reference sections of articles returned by the search processes were also examined manually for further sources. In addition to journals and conference proceedings, frequently cited textbooks in computing and health informatics experimentation were consulted (138, 152, 153). All literature sources were in English and searches performed in English.

The literature search yielded 40 publications that were used as the basis of the MICE index. 24 computing, 3 health informatics and 13 medical sources were analysed for information relating to experimental concepts, quality and/or scale items. Table 3 shows the list of sources.

A second literature review was performed just prior to the commencement of writing up the findings of this research in order to assess whether the state of informatics scales had changed. This yielded another health informatics scale (135, 154). By a manual examination of the reference

AMIA Annual Fall Symposium Proceedings
AMIA Annual Symposium Proceedings
Artificial Intelligence in Medicine
BMC Medical Informatics and Decision Making
Computer Methods and Programs in Biomedicine (including the former Computer Programs in Biomedicine)
Computers in Biology and Medicine
Computers Informatics Nursing (including the former Computers in Nursing)
Critical Reviews in Medical Informatics
Health Communication and Informatics
Health Informatics Journal
Health Information Systems and Telemedicine
International Journal of Biomedical Computing
International Journal of Clinical Monitoring and Computing
International Journal of Medical Informatics
Journal of Biomedical Informatics (including the former Computers and Biomedical Research)
Journal of Clinical Monitoring and Computing
Journal of Medical Systems
Journal of Telemedicine and Telecare
Journal of the American Medical Informatics Association
MD Computing
Medical and Biological Engineering and Computing
Medical Decision Making
Medical Informatics
Medical Informatics and the Internet in Medicine
Medinfo
Methods of Information in Medicine (including supplements)
Proceedings of the Annual Symposium on Computer Applications in Medical Care
Studies in Health Technology and Informatics
Telemedicine Journal and E-health

Table 2. Health informatics journal and conference proceedings searched in the literature review.

section of (135), another health informatics scale was discovered (150). Both scales were published prior to the first literature review and were missed using the bibliographic search strategy. Both scales were still examined and are discussed below with the results of the first literature review.

3.2.2. Analysis of Literature

When health informatics literature is examined, the overlap between it and medicine, in terms of experimental methodology, becomes clear and reaffirms the observations stated in Chapter 1 about the influence of biomedicine. Anecdotally, many evaluation researchers in health informatics have backgrounds in clinical trials and other clinical evaluation methodologies, such as case control and cohort studies. Therefore, much of health informatics methodology is based on clinical methodology. The literature on health informatics scales is testament to this, as discussed later. This may be a reason why few health informatics sources were found using the literature search strategy. Perhaps it is assumed or expected that health informatics experimenters have received adequate training through biomedical education. For instance, no step-by-step guides on experimentation were found in journals or conference proceedings, while several were discovered in computer science (15, 20-24). Despite the large overlap, it is still important to remember that there are issues in that appear particularly often in health informatics experimentation, such as contamination and difficulty of blinding. Health informatics experimentation is not an exact clone of clinical experimentation.

The literature search in computer science shows that experimentation is mostly focussed on software engineering methodology, i.e. using experimentation to assess the methods used to create software. There are fewer experiments on the benefits of information and computing technologies on human activities compared to health informatics, where most experimentation is focussed on summative assessment of health worker performance or patient outcomes. Most guidelines in computing experimentation are found in software engineering.

When reviewing health informatics experimentation, it is observed that health informatics is much more closely related to medicine than computer science. The historical and cultural reasons were discussed in Chapter 1. A good example of where health informatics is closer to medicine is in the principle of analysis by intention to treat; the concept does not exist in computing experimentation, since it is originally a medical idea. It has been adopted in health informatics as "analysis by intention to provide information." (138) (p.217) The aims of intention to treat analysis are that bias is not introduced, and interventions are seen in their "average light". People may take their new medication/use the new information resource as directed or not, and this is the real effect investigators should be measuring. Indeed, as Henneckens et al argue, investigators actually are assessing the benefit of the *offering* of an intervention because it is on this basis that randomisation occurs (155) (p. 207) rather than on the basis of full treatment compliance. They go as far to state, "Once randomized, always analyzed." (p. 207). However, the issue of how to address the effect of treatment compliance on data analysis is the opposite in computer science, i.e. consider data from non-compliant subjects as invalid and remove them from analysis. Not surprisingly, effect sizes can be inflated or become statistically significant, e.g. (156, 157). Another example is the strong desirability for random allocation that has been transferred from medicine to health informatics. The computer science experimental guidelines are less strenuous in their endorsement of random assignment.

3.2.3. Problems with Informatics Scales

Scales for measuring controlled experimental quality in informatics are few. There are no published scales in the computer science literature, and the handful from health informatics has methodological problems. Balas et al (146) published a 20-item scale in 1995 to score "health services research trials" between 0-100 points. It is unclear what was considered a health service but

Primary author (reference)	Year	Publication type	Information type
Computer science			
Basili V (158)	1986	Journal paper	Guideline
Basili V (159)	1999	Journal paper	Guideline
Boudreau M (160)	2001	Journal paper	Guideline
Brooks R (161)	1980	Journal paper	Guideline
Fenton N (16)	1994	Journal paper	Guideline
Host M (162)	2005	Conference paper	Guideline
Jarvenpaa S (163)	1985	Journal paper	Guideline
Jedlitschka A (113)	2004	Conference paper	Guideline
Juristo N (152)	2001	Textbook	Guideline
Juristo N (164)	2004	Journal paper	Guideline
Kitchenham B (122)	2002	Journal paper	Guideline
Kitchenham B (165)	2006	Conference paper	Guideline
Lott C (166)	1996	Journal paper	Guideline
Moher T (100)	1981	Conference paper	Guideline
Moher T (80)	1982	Journal paper	Guideline
Pfleeger S (167)	1995	Journal paper	Guideline
Pfleeger S (168)	1995	Journal paper	Guideline
Pfleeger S (169)	1995	Journal paper	Guideline
Pfleeger S (170)	1995	Journal paper	Guideline
Sadler C (123)	1996	Journal paper	Guideline
Singer J (114)	1999	Conference paper	Guideline
Sjoberg D (94)	2002	Conference paper	Guideline
Weinberg (119)	1998	Textbook	Guideline
Wohlin C (153)	2000	Textbook	Guideline
Health informatics			
Balas E (146)	1995	Journal paper	Scale
Johnston M (171)	1994	Journal paper	Scale
Friedman C (138)	2006	Textbook	Guideline
Medicine			
Altman D (108)	2001	Journal paper	Guideline
Chalmers I (172)	1990	Journal paper	Scale
Chalmers T (142)	1981	Journal paper	Scale
Cho M (173)	1994	Journal paper	Scale
Colditz G (174)	1989	Journal paper	Scale
Detsky A (175)	1992	Journal paper	Scale
Evans M (176)	1985	Journal paper	Scale
Goodman S (143)	1994	Journal paper	Scale
Imperiale T (177)	1990	Journal paper	Scale
Jadad A (141)	1996	Journal paper	Scale
Kleijnen J (178)	1991	Journal paper	Scale
Reisch J (179)	1989	Journal paper	Scale
Verhagen A (180)	1998	Journal paper	Scale

Table 3. List of sources critically analysed as the basis of the MICE index.

information systems were included under a criterion of "information management intervention". Being based on clinical trial method literature, it was undifferentiated from pure clinical trial scales. Experimental quality was undefined.

The scale's reliability was reported as Cohen's kappa (0.94) between two raters' final scores on a sample of studies. The authors cited Cohen's original paper (181). However, kappa, as originally described, assumes nominal data (46-48). Alternatively, weighted kappa can be used for discrete interval data and ordinal data. How Balas et al applied kappa to the final scores of the two raters was unclear and casts doubt on their scale's reliability. Validity was untested.

Balas et al's scoring scheme is hard to justify and completely arbitrary. For example, the item inquiring about randomisation can award a maximum of 10 points (if central or computerised randomisation was used) while most other items award a maximum of 2-5 points. This reflects the importance of randomisation, but on what empirical basis was this weight chosen? The rationale for the point spread between adjacent responses is also difficult to understand. For example, the item inquiring about "Definition of Sampling" requires 5 points to be given if "Entry/rejection criteria and population represented", 2 points given if "One of the above", and 0 points if "None of the above". There is distance of 3 points between two criteria stated and one stated, but there is a distance of 2 points between one and none. Different items have different spreads between steps, with a range being adopted e.g. 0-1-2, 0-1-3, 0-2-3, 0-2-5, 0-3-10. In general, scales assume that the point difference between each adjacent response is equal (182) (p. 68). It is already a significant assumption that distance between responses is interval, as mentioned in Chapter 2. There should be a good (empirical) rationale for deviating from assuming equal point spreads.

An instrument was created by McMaster University for reviewing the quality of summative trials of clinical decision support systems and was used in 3 reviews published in 1994, 1998 and 2005 (112, 171, 183). It was a 5-item scale with a possible score of 0 to 10. The authors did not describe how the scale was created i.e. from what sources, their definition of experimental quality, reliability and validity testing etc. Its soundness as a measurement tool is unclear. The review series again indicates the strong influence medicine has on health informatics evaluation and experimentation, as the authors were based in university medical departments.

The scale by Van der Loo (150) was not detected as part of the initial literature search and therefore not incorporated into the development of the MICE index. Van der Loo used a 19-item instrument to assess a variety of health informatics evaluation study designs (such as before-after, time series and fully randomised controlled experiments). It was based on principles of clinical trial conduct and, like the McMaster scale, was not developed or tested according to psychometric theory or techniques. Therefore, the discovery of this scale at the second literature review did not invalidate the need for a reliable and valid scale for informatics controlled experiments.

The second scale not detected by the initial search was created by De Keizer and Ammenwerth (135, 154). They developed a scale to rate the quality of all types of evaluation studies, such as qualitative case studies and longitudinal descriptive studies (154), not just controlled experiments.

The scale contains 10 items, each scored from 0 to 2. It was based on mostly clinical literature, e.g. CONSORT. The items inquire about high-level properties of evaluation studies. Their instrument did not influence the need for the MICE index, since their focus is not on experimentation per se. Furthermore, four main problems exist with this scale.

The first problem was that the definition of quality was confused and not highly useful because of the broad scope of the scale. Quality was defined as report quality rather than of the study itself (184), yet some items addressed methodological appropriateness, e.g. "Methods seem adequate to answer study questions". Final scores may be difficult to interpret and hard to use. Evaluative studies performed appropriately within the confines of their possible rigor could have the same score but are of different strengths in terms of establishing cause and effect. There is, by design, less confidence in the results of an uncontrolled before-after study than a randomised controlled trial, yet both could have the same score. If keeping to a definition of report quality, a high score tells the reader the paper has been written well. However, a more informative use is the assessment of confidence of prediction and strength of results. This is particularly important if quality is to be used in meta-analysis.

This problem relates to defining quality as merely the clarity of the study report. This is indeed important since an unclear report makes interpreting the results of a study difficult. However, alone, it is insufficient in determining the usefulness (quality) of a study. A method may be explained well but completely wrong insofar as testing a hypothesis. Therefore, a scale that measures report quality, especially one that encompasses all types of evaluative studies, is difficult to apply with meaningful results.

The second problem relates to the item, "Any comparison that is done between groups is fair." As the authors indicate (184), not every evaluative study may compare groups, therefore the item could become impossible to answer. It is unclear how to deal with this situation with regards to scoring.

The third problem is possibly reliability. Kappa was measured between 2 raters for each item using 9 studies (range = 0.53 - 1, averaged kappa over 10 items = 0.87). It is unclear whether unweighted or weighted kappa was used. Only the latter can be used for ordinal or discrete interval data. Finally, testing 9 studies was probably too few for a confident estimate of reliability (138) (p. 126).

The fourth problem is validity, which was not tested; this was acknowledged by the authors (184).

In summary, no scales for measuring the quality of controlled experiments exist in the computer science literature, and those in the health informatics literature were inadequate due to psychometric problems. Formal validity testing was a glaring omission.

59

3.2.4. Definition of Experimental Quality and Scope

The definition of experimental quality was derived from the literature sources. There was little consensus on what aspects of an experiment determine good quality. Even among the medical scales, less than 25% defined what quality meant (109). Moher et al put forward their definition as "the confidence that the trial design, conduct, and analysis has minimized or avoided biases in its treatment comparisons." (109) Furthermore, they distinguished between the quality of the method and the quality of the study report. The definition used for the development of the MICE index was that an experiment should have high internal and high external validity (a good experiment affords confident prediction), and its report should be comprehensible. Put simply, an experiment's results should be correct, useful to the reader's own situation and understandable. This definition is similar to Moher et al's but considers the importance of good reporting. An experiment may be performed well, but if it is poorly communicated then the results become questionable or useless, and replication of the study becomes difficult or impossible. This definition was used to pool experimental concepts and develop questionnaire items.

The scope of the scale was defined a priori. The MICE index is defined for controlled experiments in computer science and health informatics and that involve human subjects. It can be used for summative and formative experiments. It cannot be used for other empirical study designs, e.g. case studies. Control groups can be concurrent or historical, within subject (crossover) or between subjects. Treatments can be compared to no treatment or other standards and may consist of informatics objects (such as information systems or paper-based tools) or human-based methods (such as software and interface development). Potentially, any human-based informatics experiments can be assessed with the MICE index, e.g. whether a clinical information system improves diagnostic ability, protocol adherence or patient or resource outcomes; whether groups or individuals are better at detecting software faults; whether computer-supported collaborative work improves the performance of workers; whether the format of presented information affects decision making. The index requires users to have knowledge of experimental design, statistical methods and informatics methods and tools. Users will most likely be empirical researchers in informatics.

3.3. Item Generation

3.3.1. Pooling of Items and Concepts

The 40 publication sources from the first literature search were read and summarised to pool pre-existing items and experimental concepts. As each source was summarised, experimental concepts were listed in a spreadsheet (Microsoft Excel 2000, Microsoft, Seattle, USA) against the source.

Some concepts were similar in nature or expressed in synonymous ways by different sources. Some concepts were related by different levels of abstraction, i.e. a concept could be hierarchical to another, e.g. appropriate use of statistical methods subsumes use of confidence levels. When developing the spreadsheet table, sources were deemed to support a concept if the source directly reiterated it or the wording had the same semantic meaning. Hierarchical concepts were kept as individual concepts or else the problem of all concepts being subsumed by a few with loss of detail would have occurred. The issue of the level of abstraction of guidelines has been noted by Kitchenham et al (122). As each source was summarised, concepts were added to the table or sources were entered against already existing concepts. The process of adding concepts was permissive, rather than to force concepts together or force sources to support an individual concept. The rationale was that this stage was not meant to be strict and quantitative but rather to brainstorm the area of experimental quality and gather an informal consensus. This would help to establish content validity. After the 40th source was analysed, the summaries were analysed again to ensure that concepts added after earlier sources were checked against them. Each source was checked against each concept and each concept checked against each source. The data is shown in Appendix A. Concepts are listed under broad experimental sections (Introduction, Method, Study Design etc). Some organisation and re-wording of concepts were required to clarify meaning. Therefore, concepts are not necessarily taken verbatim. However, some concepts are almost identical to the original source.

Over 200 experimental concepts were produced. Some are not highly distinct from others, and the decision that a concept should exist separately from others or that a concept was endorsed by a source was subjective. This stage also permitted inclusion of concepts that were clearly not related to quality as defined, since the decision to include a concept as a questionnaire item came later. For instance, some researchers feel it is necessary to give feedback to participants about how they performed at the end of an experiment. This concept is unlikely to affect quality as defined for the MICE index.

3.3.2. Selection of Experimental Concepts

The permissive nature of the item and concept pooling provided a wide view of experimentation in computer science, health informatics and medicine. Not all concepts were included in the MICE questionnaire.

The choice of concepts to be used for item questions was based on several subjective criteria. The frequency of endorsement of concepts by sources was done by visual approximation of the spreadsheet ("eyeballing"), rather than using a frequency distribution, because it was acknowledged that there is ambiguity in wording and hierarchy of concepts. Precise counts therefore were unjustified. Important selection criteria were the author's knowledge of experimental theory and evidence of experimental conduct on quality, e.g. while allocation concealment is not recognised specifically in computer science guidelines, there is empirical evidence that it can affect the credibility of results (see Chapter 4.) The choice of concepts was also based on the definitions of quality and scope for the MICE index. For instance, ethical issues, while important for other reasons, do not impact on experimental quality as defined. Many of the medical concepts were not within the scope of the index, e.g. use of identical placebo and measuring the bioavailability of treatments (concepts related to drug therapies). For some concepts, it was also impossible to establish compliance or the outcomes. For example, Wohlin recommends accounting for random irrelevancies that disturb the experimental environment (153) (p. 68). This could affect internal validity but how could the index user judge this concept? If there were unexpected events that affected validity, then the study could be marked down. If there were not any such events, was it because none really occurred or because the authors neglected to report them? This is similar to the concept of attempting to record side effects of a treatment. If no information about side effects is reported, the case of absent side effects cannot be distinguished from side effects not being monitored. Thus, from a quality point of view, it might be good that no side effects occurred but bad that the investigators did not try to monitor them. Another example is trying to avoid participants who are biased for or against a treatment. This cannot be known as it involves asking participants, who would presumably indicate neutrality. Hence these examples show that while certain ideas in experimental conduct and quality are important, not all are amenable to translation into scale items. Since judgements are required from the index user, concepts translated into questionnaire items must be "answerable".

3.3.3. Item Writing and Format

The translation of experimental concepts to item questions and format followed the general principles in Chapter 2.

Some items were necessarily dichotomous, such as whether a statistician was consulted and presence of unit of analysis error. Most items were recognised to be continuous. Most of the responses were treated on a 7-point scale. While there is no direct evidence that experimental quality can be distinguished at any number of levels, Miller's work provides some basis for using 7 response steps of discrimination (144).

Items were written at an appropriate reading level for the intended users. Care was taken to minimise ambiguity of items, including providing information where needed to answer items.

Either a unipolar or bipolar format could have been used. A unipolar format was chosen to reflect "amounts" of quality (low to high). However, Likert-type formats, where users agree or disagree with declarative statements on quality, might be equivalent; this is yet unknown.

3.3.4. Item Scoring

The scoring system was devised in the fashion of Cho (173). Each item's value is determined by the response alternative. The lowest alternative (indicating poor quality) has a value of 0, and each successive alternative (indicating better quality) is incremented by 1. The maximum value for an item is between 1 and 6. Inapplicable items are not scored. The scale's final score is calculated as the total of all the item values divided by the total possible score (i.e. excluding the NA items). This gives a final score of between 0 and 1 regardless of item applicability and allows comparison between different experiments. All items are equally weighted. The rationale for equal weighting is two-fold. Firstly, there is not enough empirical basis for the degree to which certain experimental mistakes affect the quality (credibility) of results. As mentioned above, on what basis did Balas decide that randomisation should have an influence on the final score several times that of other items? It appears that weighting for the Balas scale and quality scales in general is mostly arbitrary. Secondly, as described in Chapter 2, sufficiently large scales are less affected by weighting.

It was defined for some items that if a study report provided insufficient information to be able to answer the item, quality would be considered as poor. For instance, outcome assessors should be blinded to whether an outcome comes from a treatment or control group. If the study authors do not describe assessor blinding, it is equivalent to not having been done, even if it was actually performed in the experiment but simply neglected in the report. This is consistent with the definition of experimental quality, since the lack of certain important information makes findings questionable.

Another related issue was how to consider study reports that cite further information about an experiment in other publications. This often happens when measurement methods are described in another paper and the main experimental report cites that paper instead of repeating those results. It was defined a priori that a paper should be a complete enough account of an experiment to allow readers to judge whether the findings are credible and applicable. Hence the MICE index would still penalise a report even if methodological issues were better described in other reports.

3.3.5. Item Review

An early draft of scale items was reviewed by a statistician experienced in experimentation. The outcomes of this process were subjective recommendations by the expert. Some items were modified (data not shown.)

3.3.6.   MICE-80 Questionnaire

At the end of item creation, an initial prototype questionnaire containing 80 items was ready for reliability and validity tests. This is the MICE-80 index. The MICE-38 index is the more efficient version and is the subject of Chapter 4. However, the MICE-80 items that were removed to produce the 38-item version can be found in Appendix B.

3.4.   Statistical Methods for Reliability and Validity Tests

All reliability and validity statistical tests were performed with SPSS version 15 (SPSS, Chicago, USA). As elaborated later, MICE scores were tested for normality using the Shapiro-Wilks test, measures of skewness and kurtosis, as well as plotted on histograms and Q-Q plots.

T-tests were accompanied by Wilcoxon rank sum tests, and Pearson correlations by Spearman rho correlation. For t-tests, variances were not assumed to be equal, and thus Levene's test was applied. All statistical significance tests were considered significant at a p value less than 0.05.

3.5.   MICE-80 Reliability Tests

The MICE-80 questionnaire was tested for reliability with the test-retest method using the author as the rater. Reports of controlled experiments in computer science and health informatics were chosen as test studies. For computer science studies, the ACM Digital Library database was searched for "controlled experiment". Returned references were selected based on whether they were reports of an actual experiment and then on coin toss. 25 such studies were selected. For health informatics studies, the review of Garg et al (McMaster University) (112) was used. This often-cited review examined 100 controlled trials of clinical decision support systems. Trials were marked on paper slips, which were then drawn from a hat. 33 such trials from Garg et al were selected. When any study was not obtainable in full text through the University of Western Sydney library, another was selected using the above processes. In total, 58 controlled experimental studies were used to test the MICE index's reliability. At least 30 to 50 studies were considered needed, to permit further statistical analysis based on central limit theorem (182) (p. 222), (185) (p. 90), (186) (p. 229). Table 4 and Table 5 show the list of test studies. Most experiments in computer science were assessments of software engineering methods. The selection of health informatics experiments was biased towards summative evaluation of informatics tools because of the nature of the review, but this is probably representative of many experiments conducted in health informatics.

Primary author	Year	Experiment assessed effect of:
Computer science		
Ali Babar (187)	2006	Providing software change categories on the quality of scenario profiles.
Ali Babar (188)	2006	Distributed meetings on the quality of scenario profiles.
Anda (189)	2003	Use case vs. responsibility-driven methods on object oriented design
Arisholm (190)	2001	Responsibility-driven vs. mainframe designs on software changeability.
Briand (157)	2001	Object-oriented principles effects on software comprehension and changeability.
Bunse (191)	2006	A method for translating UML models to source code on software comprehension and verification.
Canfora (192)	2006	Test-driven development on software testing quality.
Golden (193)	2005	Usability-supporting architectural patterns for software architecture design on modification tasks.
Hu (194)	2006	Metamorphic testing on fault detection.
Johnson (195)	1997	Review meetings on software testing.
Lopes (196)	1993	A software tool for debugging Ada programmes on fault detection programme comprehension.
Lott (197)	1997	Online process guidance on software development.
Muller (198)	2005	Pair programming vs. peer review on software quality and cost.
Myers (199)	1978	Several of types of fault detection methods.
Myrtveit (156)	1999	A software tool and a regression model for estimating software project costs.
Ng (200)	2006	Refactoring on the maintenance of software.
Prechelt (201)	1998	Type checking on fault detection.
Prechelt (202)	2001	Design patterns on software maintenance.
Prechelt (203)	2002	Design pattern documentation on software maintenance.
Prechelt (204)	2003	Inheritance depth on software maintenance.
Sears (205)	1994	Split menus on usability.
Sonnenwald (206)	2003	A scientific collaboratory system on research work quality.
Vokac (207)	2004	Design patterns on software maintenance.
Wojcicki (208)	2006	A software tool and code inspection on fault detection.
Zettel (209)	2005	Different information support on a CASE tool's usability.

Table 4. List of controlled experimental studies in computer science used to test index reliability.

Test-retest was applied in 3 rounds. Each of the 58 studies was assessed with the 80-item questionnaire. Each round took approximately 3-4 weeks. Studies were assessed in the same order hence the interval between assessing the same study was approximately 3-4 weeks. This is considered sufficient time to prevent serious memory effects (131) (p. 137), (210). A spreadsheet (Excel 2000, Microsoft, Seattle, USA) was created to store the individual item values and to automate calculation of final scores. Final scores were not calculated until the last study of round 3 was completed. In addition, as soon as each study was assessed, all item results were hidden using the column hiding function of Excel 2000. These measures aided prevention of memory effects. The only memory effects to have occurred were those of being familiar with the content of a paper and not the individual item responses. 3 rounds were chosen instead of the usual 2 rounds (test and a single retest) to improve the estimate of reliability (138) (p. 125). Reliability was calculated as an intraclass correlation coefficient (ICC) using a two way random effects model, absolute agreement and single measures. This was based on analysis of variance (ANOVA) of the final MICE scores between rounds and between studies. A two-way random effects model was appropriate because the author assessed all studies and was considered to be a random sample of all possible raters (131) (p. 134). Because the value of a study's final score should be similar with each round rather than simple ranking, absolute agreement rather than consistency was applied (211). Finally, single measure reliability was used since individual scores were the unit of analysis (211).

Primary author	Year	Experiment assessed effect of:
Health informatics		
Bonevski (212)	1999	A reminder information system on preventative health measures.
Brownbridge (213)	1986	A computerised protocol on management of hypertension.
Cannon (214)	2000	A reminder information system on mental health screening rates.
Christakis (215)	2001	An information system on correct antibiotic prescribing.
Demakis (216)	2000	A reminder information system on management tasks for common health problems.
Dexter (217)	1998	A reminder information system on completion of advance directives.
Fitzmaurice (218)	1996	A decision support system on management of anticoagulation.
Fitzmaurice (219)	2000	A decision support system on management of anticoagulation.
Gonzalez (220)	1989	A decision support system for dosing of aminophylline.
Hickling (221)	1989	A decision support system for dosing of aminoglycosides.
Horn (222)	2002	A decision support system for prescribing parenteral nutrition for neonates.
Kuperman (223)	1999	An alerting laboratory information system on clinician response time.
Lewis (224)	1996	A mental health assessment tool on mental health outcomes.
Lowensteyn (225)	1998	Computerised risk profiles on coronary risk outcomes.
Mazzuca (226)	1990	A reminder information system on diabetic management.
McAlister (227)	1986	Computerised protocol and feedback on hypertension management.
McDonald (228)	1984	A reminder information system on management tasks for common health problems.
Poller (229)	1998	A decision support system on management of anticoagulation.
Rosser (230)	1991	A reminder information system on preventative health measures.
Rossi (231)	1997	A reminder information system on incorrect antihypertensive prescribing.
Rotman (232)	1996	A prescribing system on costs and drug interactions.
Ryff-de Leche (233)	1992	Diabetes monitoring systems on diabetic control.
Schriger (234)	2001	A mental health diagnostic system on mental health management.
Selker (235)	1998	A cardiac ischaemia diagnostic system on appropriate triage.
Tamblyn (236)	2003	A decision support system on inappropriate prescribing.
Tang (237)	1999	A reminder information system on influenza vaccination.
Thomas (238)	1983	An audit system on health care costs.
Tierney (239)	1993	An ordering information system on health care costs.
Vadher (240)	1997	A decision support system on management of anticoagulation.
Vadher (241)	1997	A decision support system on management of anticoagulation.
Verner (242)	1992	A decision support system for dosing of theophylline.
Wexler (243)	1975	Accuracy of a paediatric diagnostic system.
Young (244)	1981	A reminder information system on management tasks for common health problems.

Table 5. List of controlled experimental studies in health informatics used to test index reliability.

The final scores for each study, per round, are shown in Table 6, which is in the form of an objects-by-observations matrix (see Chapter 1), and summary statistics are shown in Table 7. The raw data of individual item responses for each study per round is not produced in this book due to space (the worksheet contains nearly 14000 cells: 80 items x 3 rounds x 58 studies) but may be obtained from the author for examination.

66

Computer science	Rnd 1	Rnd 2	Rnd 3	Health Informatics	Rnd 1	Rnd 2	Rnd 3
Ali Babar (187)	.599	.647	.631	Bonevski (212)	.635	.629	.643
Ali Babar (188)	.636	.669	.648	Brownbridge (213)	.438	.396	.436
Anda (189)	.524	.524	.515	Cannon (214)	.590	.498	.508
Arisholm (190)	.504	.496	.501	Christakis (215)	.663	.692	.683
Briand (157)	.598	.642	.619	Demakis (216)	.644	.646	.638
Bunse (191)	.596	.645	.642	Dexter (217)	.599	.601	.589
Canfora (192)	.603	.638	.626	Fitzmaurice (218)	.426	.398	.404
Golden (193)	.514	.547	.535	Fitzmaurice (219)	.559	.538	.553
Hu (194)	.389	.435	.407	Gonzalez (220)	.570	.593	.575
Johnson (195)	.582	.573	.585	Hickling (221)	.580	.571	.565
Lopes (196)	.416	.454	.448	Horn (222)	.388	.385	.406
Lott (197)	.611	.599	.597	Kuperman (223)	.578	.535	.541
Muller (198)	.546	.598	.565	Lewis (224)	.537	.581	.593
Myers (199)	.509	.552	.528	Lowensteyn (225)	.548	.604	.608
Myrtveit (156)	.451	.545	.519	Mazzuca (226)	.585	.694	.668
Ng (200)	.521	.521	.512	McAlister (227)	.679	.724	.691
Prechelt (201)	.481	.510	.484	McDonald (228)	.506	.650	.612
Prechelt (202)	.463	.521	.506	Poller (229)	.599	.620	.633
Prechelt (203)	.540	.534	.537	Rosser (230)	.516	.612	.599
Prechelt (204)	.519	.554	.543	Rossi (231)	.755	.745	.705
Sears (205)	.493	.548	.534	Rotman (232)	.701	.738	.729
Sonnenwald (206)	.696	.729	.717	Ryff-de Leche (233)	.540	.518	.550
Vokac (207)	.564	.553	.544	Schriger (234)	.783	.803	.809
Wojcicki (208)	.517	.551	.539	Selker (235)	.772	.762	.777
Zettel (209)	.602	.596	.599	Tamblyn (236)	.770	.765	.743
				Tang (237)	.476	.549	.525
				Thomas (238)	.498	.505	.508
				Tierney (239)	.605	.608	.602
				Vadher (240)	.716	.699	.706
				Vadher (241)	.534	.575	.558
				Verner (242)	.539	.545	.558
				Wexler (243)	.346	.420	.404
				Young (244)	.336	.410	.407

Table 6. Test studies' MICE-80 scores produced during assessment of test-retest reliability.
Rnd: round.

	Round 1	Round 2	Round 3
N	58	58	58
Mean	.560	.583	.576
Median	.554	.574	.565
Standard deviation	.100	.098	.094
Skewness	.146	.082	.189
Standard error of skewness	.314	.314	.314
Kurtosis	.174	-.197	-.048
Standard error of kurtosis	.618	.618	.618

Table 7. Summary statistics from test-retest reliability assessment of MICE-80.

Table 8 shows the results of the analysis of variance calculations. The ICC was based on the formulae modified from (131) (p. 134):

$$ICC = \frac{\sigma^2_{studies}}{\sigma^2_{studies} + \sigma^2_{raters} + \sigma^2_{error}}$$

$$ICC = \frac{MS_{studies} - MS_{error}}{MS_{studies} + \frac{k}{n}(MS_{raters} - MS_{error}) + (k-1)MS_{error}}$$

where σ^2 is the variance, MS is the mean square, k is the number of raters (i.e. 1) and n is the number of studies. The reliability of the MICE-80 questionnaire was 0.935 (95% CI 0.884 - 0.962).

		Sum of squares	df	Mean square	F	p
Between Studies		1.562	57	.027		
Within Studies	Between Rounds	.016	2	.008	15.462	.000
	Residual	.057	114	.001		
	Total	.073	116	.001		
Total		1.635	173	.009		
ICC .935 (95% CI .884 - .962)						

Table 8. ANOVA and ICC results for MICE-80 scores in Table 6.

3.6. MICE-80 Normality Tests

There were 2 purposes for analysing the normality of MICE scores. There is no empirical evidence of the distributional nature of experimental quality in informatics. Secondly, for statistical test constraints, it is useful to know whether data is normal.

Prior to performing parametric validity tests, the MICE-80 scores in Table 6 were assessed for normality by examining data skewness and kurtosis, histograms, Q-Q plots and carrying out the Shapiro-Wilks test. Skewness and kurtosis for each round were almost zero, supporting normality (see Table 7.) In particular, the ratio of skewness and kurtosis to their standard errors was between - 2 and 2 (SPSS version 15, SPSS, Chicago, USA). Histograms in Figure 3 showed approximately bell-shaped curves.

When scores from all rounds were pooled, the distribution remained near normal. Skewness was 0.123 (standard error = 0.184), and kurtosis was −0.080 (standard error = 0.366). Figure 4 shows the histogram and normal Q-Q plot of all scores. Again, a bell-shaped curved is evident, and the Q-Q plot has little deviance. The Shapiro-Wilks test on all rounds was not significant and therefore further supported normality (Shapiro-Wilks statistic = 0.985, df = 174, p = 0.063).

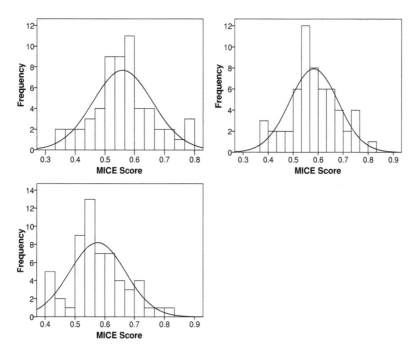

Figure 3. Histogram of MICE-80 scores produced during round 1 (top left), 2 (top right) and 3 of reliability assessment.

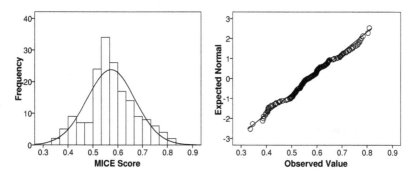

Figure 4. Histogram (left) and normal Q-Q plot of MICE-80 scores produced during reliability assessment (all rounds).

Distributions of samples involved in t-testing (convergent validity tests [statistician assistance, see p. 76] and known-groups tests [dichotomisation by McMaster University score, see p. 74]) were also examined to ensure that samples were similar and normal (245) (p. 493) . Distributions of the statistician-assisted and unassisted samples were examined including and excluding adjustment for items inquiring about statistical assistance (see p. 76.) The statistician-assisted sample was approximately normal as shown in Table 9, Figure 5 and Figure 6. The unassisted sample was not normally distributed (Table 9, Figure 7 and Figure 8) but did not strongly deviate from normal.

	Statistician-assisted sample	Statistician-unassisted sample
Including item		
Skewness (SE)	-.838 (.536)	.276 (.374)
Kurtosis (SE)	.592 (1.038)	2.058 (.733)*
Shapiro-Wilks statistic	.947	.934
Shapiro-Wilks df	18	40
Shapiro-Wilks p	.381	.023*
Excluding item		
Skewness (SE)	-.839 (.536)	.279 (.374)
Kurtosis (SE)	.595 (1.038)	2.063 (.733)*
Shapiro-Wilks statistic	.947	.935
Shapiro-Wilks df	18	40
Shapiro-Wilks p	.380	.023*

Table 9. Normality statistics for samples used in MICE-80 convergent construct validity tests (samples with and without statistical assistance).

*: non-normality; SE: standard error.

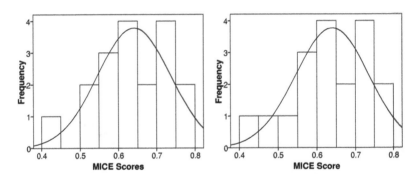

Figure 5. Histogram of MICE-80 scores for the statistician-assisted sample including (left) and excluding the item inquiring about assistance (see p. 76.)

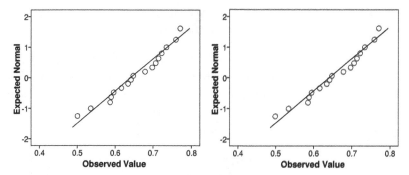

Figure 6. Normal Q-Q plots of MICE-80 scores for the statistician-assisted sample including (left) and excluding the item inquiring about assistance (see p. 76.)

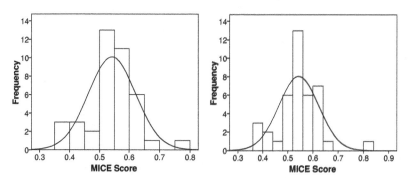

Figure 7. Histograms of MICE-80 scores for the statistician-unassisted sample including (left) and excluding the item inquiring about assistance (see p. 76.)

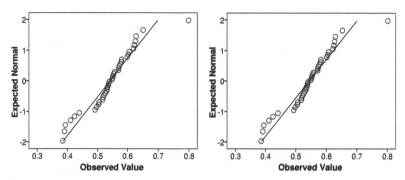

Figure 8. Normal Q-Q plots of MICE-80 scores for the statistician-unassisted sample including (left) and excluding the item inquiring about assistance (see p. 76.)

Distributions of samples dichotomised according to McMaster University score (see p. 74) were approximately normal as shown in Table 10, Figure 9 and Figure 10.

With regards to statistical testing, a conservative approach of using both nonparametric and parametric tests was adopted (152). While the analysis of all scores suggests experimental quality is normal, there is not yet an accumulated body of evidence to support normality of controlled experiment quality in informatics. Furthermore, some sample sizes were small (N < 15) and unequal, which favour the use of nonparametric tests (245) (p. 493).

	McMaster score <6	McMaster score >=6
Skewness (SE)	1.132 (.687)	-.042 (.481)
Kurtosis (SE)	1.704 (1.334)	.400 (.935)
Shapiro-Wilks statistic	.875	.968
Shapiro-Wilks df	10	23
Shapiro-Wilks p	.114	.636

Table 10. Normality statistics for samples used in MICE-80 known-groups criterion validity tests (dichotomised into samples of high and low quality studies).

SE: standard error.

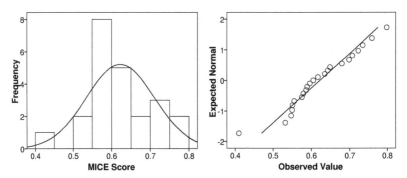

Figure 9. Histogram (left) and normal Q-Q plot of MICE-80 scores dichotomised according the McMaster scale as high quality studies (score >=6) (see p. 74.)

3.7. MICE-80 Validity Tests

Face and content validity were not formally tested. Because the MICE index was developed from experimental literature of 3 fields (computer science, health informatics and medicine), with statistical expert help and contained a large number of items, face and content validity was assumed. Furthermore, these forms of validity are less useful than criterion and construct validity (138) (p. 132), therefore only criterion and construct validity were formally measured.

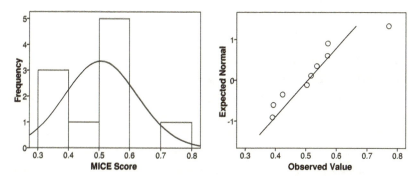

Figure 10. Histogram (left) and normal Q-Q plot of MICE-80 scores dichotomised according the McMaster scale as low quality studies (score <6) (see p. 74.)

3.7.1. Criterion Validity by Known-Groups and Journal Impact Factor

It is difficult to apply criterion validity when gold standards do not exist. Since there are no other reliable and valid instruments to measure the MICE index against, a known-groups approach and a related standard were used. The known-groups method required that the MICE index could differentiate members of one group from another (125) (p. 54). That is, could it classify poor quality studies from high quality studies? The first step required obtaining experimental studies of good and poor quality, as judged by another standard. One option was to provide a sample of studies to a panel of experts for prospectively categorising into good and poor. Another option was to use a (systematic) review that assessed study quality (a retrospective approach). Because such reviews are often performed by panels, the two are approximately equivalent. The former option was not chosen because of limited resources; an expert panel would have needed to assess 58 publications and have been familiar with both health informatics and computer science experimentation. Time and access to such judges were problematic (this can be a focus for future research.) Instead, the Garg et al review (112) (McMaster University) was chosen as the arbiter of study quality. Each of the studies reviewed by Garg et al had been assessed with their McMaster scale. The McMaster scale was not considered satisfactory enough to have been directly used as a gold standard (i.e. applying the MICE and McMaster scales to studies and correlating the results). Instead, the McMaster scale and review were viewed as sufficient to classify at an approximate level (i.e. good versus poor) and assumed to be equivalent to an expert panel review where experts use their own critical appraisement skills. Indeed, the McMaster review may be superior than a prospective panel review where there is no attempt to measure reliability.

For the MICE index to be able to classify good and poor quality study groups, good studies should have higher MICE scores than poor studies.

The 33 health informatics studies (see Table 5) were selected again as test studies for criterion validity. They were dichotomised into good and poor quality using a threshold McMaster score of 6 points (since they had been selected from the Garg et al review, each had already been scored using the McMaster scale.) The McMaster score has a maximum value of 10 points. Studies scoring greater than or equal to 6 were defined, a priori, as good. Less than 6 were defined as poor. Next, the scores in Table 6 were averaged across rounds to produce a single MICE score for each study. Thus, a set of MICE scores for the high quality group and a set of MICE scores for the poor quality group were produced. The mean MICE scores for the good and poor groups were analysed for difference using a 2-tailed independent samples t-test and Wilcoxon rank sum test (the null hypothesis being that the 2 means were from the same population of quality).

At no point did the McMaster scores influence the MICE scores produced during reliability testing as the rater was blinded to the McMaster score. This was achieved by avoidance of looking at the McMaster score when test studies were selected and assessed. Without such blinding, assessment using the MICE index could have been consciously or unconsciously correlated with the McMaster score, which would artificially strengthen the relationship between MICE scores and dichotomised studies.

Only health informatics studies were used for criterion validity testing because there were no reviews in the computer science literature that quantitatively assessed or categorised controlled experiments as the Garg et al paper did.

Table 11 and Table 12 show that the MICE-80 questionnaire differentiated between high and low quality studies. The high quality group of studies scored 0.117 points higher than poor quality group ($p = 0.004$). Levene's test was not significant indicating that equal variances could be assumed (though significance remained even with unequal variances). Table 13 shows the results of Wilcoxon rank sum test, which is also statistically significant. Results support that the MICE-80 questionnaire is criterion valid using a known-groups approach.

McMaster score	N	Mean MICE score	Standard deviation
>=6 (good quality)	23	.623	.088
<6 (poor quality)	10	.506	.119

Table 11. Descriptive statistics of MICE-80 scores dichotomised into good and poor quality group studies.

	Levene's test		t-test (2-tailed)			
	F	p	t	df	p	Mean difference (95% CI)
Equal variances assumed	.604	.443	3.140	31	.004	.117 (.041 - .192)
Equal variances not assumed			2.786	13.497	.015	.117 (.027 - .207)

Table 12. 2-tailed independent samples t-test comparing the means of MICE-80 scores from good and poor quality groups.

McMaster score	N	Mean rank	Sum of ranks
>=6 (good quality)	23	20.30	467.00
<6 (poor quality)	10	9.40	94.00
Wilcoxon W 94.00			
p (2-tailed) .003			

Table 13. Wilcoxon rank sum test comparing MICE-80 scores from good and poor quality groups.

The second approach of testing criterion validity was to use a related standard. Journal Impact Factor (JIF) (246) has been used controversially as an indicator of medical research and trial quality (247, 248). Thus, would the MICE score for a study be correlated with the paper's JIF? This question was exploratory, to see how useful JIF might be for criterion validation, rather than to obtain evidence of MICE's criterion validity. The accuracy of JIF to indicate clinical trial quality has been variable and still subject to research (249, 250). To examine the relationship, the MICE scores produced during test-retest reliability assessment were used (Table 6). They were averaged across rounds and correlated with JIF of the report's journal (see Appendix C for raw data.) JIF from 2006 were used (ISI Web of Knowledge Journal Citation Report 2006 Edition, The Thompson Corporation, Stamford, USA). 15 of the 58 studies did not have a corresponding JIF since these studies appeared in conference proceedings or the Journal Citation Report did not cover that particular journal. Pearson and Spearman rho correlation were used to assess the relationship between MICE score and JIF.

Figure 11 shows a scatterplot of JIF versus MICE score. The correlation was weak to modest (Pearson r = 0.329, 2-tailed p = 0.031, Spearman rho = 0.482, 2-tailed p = 0.001). Results do not convincingly support that JIF is a useful related standard against which to judge the MICE-80 questionnaire's validity.

The relationship of MICE score to JIF should be interpreted with caution. JIF from both computer science (N = 13) and health informatics (N = 30) were used in analysis. While there are several semantic relationships between computer science and health informatics, this may not extend to mixing JIF from both areas. Indeed, JIF between different disciplines may not be highly comparable, particularly slowly changing fields (251). Also, JIF are not consistent (by definition they are the ratio of a current year to the previous 2 years.) The 2006 JCR edition was used, but results may have been different with previous editions.

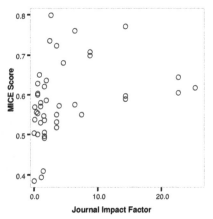

Figure 11. Scatterplot of MICE-80 scores produced during reliability assessment vs. studies' Journal Impact Factors.

3.7.2. Construct Validity

Construct validity was tested using convergent and divergent methods. The convergent hypothesis was that the help of a statistician (or equivalent expert in experimental methods, e.g. epidemiologist) would improve experimental quality. The MICE scores produced during reliability assessment (see Table 6) were again analysed. Studies were dichotomised into those where it was clear a statistician assisted and those where it was not (assumed unassisted), producing 2 sets of MICE scores. Scores for each study were averaged over the 3 rounds and compared using a 2-tailed independent samples t-test and Wilcoxon rank sum test. In addition, because one of the MICE index's items rewards points to studies when a statistician is used, scores were recalculated with this item removed before averaging over rounds and performing the inference tests again (the item was deleted from the spreadsheet used for recording responses during the test-retest assessment, and final scores automatically adjusted.) Appendix C contains the raw data of MICE scores with and without the item. Table 14 shows the mean MICE scores for statistician-assisted and unassisted studies when the item inquiring about statistical assistance is included and excluded. Whether the item is included or excluded in analysis, the effect is small (the difference between groups fell approximately 0.003 points when excluded) and did not affect statistical significance. Table 15 shows that statistical assistance improves quality by approximately 0.1 of a point (p = 0.000). Results of the Wilcoxon rank sum test are shown in Table 16 and are also statistically significant. Results support that the MICE-80 questionnaire is convergent construct valid.

	Statistician	N	Mean MICE score	Standard deviation
Item included	Yes	18	.642	.095
	No	40	.542	.079
Item excluded	Yes	18	.640	.095
	No	40	.544	.079

Table 14. Descriptive statistics of MICE-80 scores for studies where statistical assistance was provided and not provided.

Results shown for when the item inquiring about statistical assistance is included and excluded.

		Levene's test		t-test (2-tailed)			
		F	p	t	df	p	Mean difference (95% CI)
Item included	Equal variances assumed	1.241	.270	4.162	56	.000	.100 (.052 - .147)
	Equal variances not assumed			3.881	28.084	.001	.100 (.047 - .152)
Item excluded	Equal variances assumed	1.240	.270	4.040	56	.000	.097 (.049 - .145)
	Equal variances not assumed			3.767	28.073	.001	.097 (.044 - .150)

Table 15. 2-tailed independent samples t-test comparing the means of MICE-80 scores from studies that had and did not have statistician assistance.

Results shown for when the item inquiring about statistical assistance is included and excluded.

	Statistician	N	Mean rank	Sum of ranks
Item included	Yes	18	41.78	752.00
	No	40	23.98	959.00
	Wilcoxon W 959.00 p (2-tailed) .000			
Item excluded	Yes	18	41.78	752.00
	No	40	23.98	959.00
	Wilcoxon W 959.00 p (2-tailed) .000			

Table 16. Wilcoxon rank sum test comparing MICE-80 scores of studies that had and did not have statistician assistance.

Results for when the item inquiring about statistical assistance is included and excluded.

The divergent construct validity hypotheses were that experimental quality should not be related to the number of authors, pages or cited references or year of publication of a report. The hypothesis is that these variables are not likely to affect or reflect whether experiments are conducted well. Again, the MICE scores produced during reliability assessment (Table 6) were used for analysis. The MICE scores were averaged over rounds and correlated against study author, page and reference counts and year. Pearson and Spearman rho correlation were used for each relationship. Appendix C contains the raw data. Figure 12 shows the scatterplots, and Table 17 shows Pearson r and Spearman rho correlation coefficients. Correlations were weak, supporting the divergent construct hypotheses. The MICE-80 questionnaire is therefore divergent construct valid.

	N	Author	p	Page	p	Reference	p	Year	p
r	58	.171	.200	-.196	.140	.127	.343	-.170	.203
rho	58	.175	.188	-.217	.102	.119	.374	-.140	.293

Table 17. Pearson r and Spearman rho correlation between MICE-80 scores and counts of authors, pages and references and year of publication.

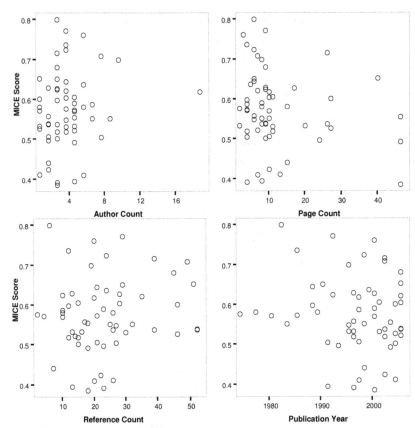

Figure 12. Scatterplots of MICE-80 scores produced during reliability assessment vs. studies' number of authors, pages, references and publication year.

In summary, the 80-item questionnaire (MICE-80) was demonstrated to be valid according to several forms of validity. It is subjectively face and content valid because it looks as if it captures controlled experimental quality; it was distilled from a large number of experimental concepts from computer science, health informatics and medicine and with expert input. More importantly, it is criterion valid against a standard of predefined poor and good quality. Also important is that it is

78

construct valid since it behaves in a way that might be expected hypothetically. That is, scores improve when statistical experts help with an experiment. Scores do not correlate with variables unlikely to affect or reflect quality (number of author investigators, page length of the report, number of cited references in the report, year of report publication).

3.8.   Item Reduction

The 80-item questionnaire (MICE-80) was demonstrated to be reliable and valid. The ICC was 0.935 (95% CI 0.884 - 0.962), and criterion and construct validity were empirically established. However, the questionnaire took 30 to 60 minutes to apply (i.e. not including report reading time) and occasionally up to 90 minutes, depending on the length and complexity of a study's report. According to the Spearman-Brown prophecy formula, halving the questionnaire length would have reduced reliability to 0.88. Since shorter scales are less burdensome on users, and there was "reliability to spare" (125) (p. 97), the 80-item questionnaire underwent item reduction.

To shorten the index, items were removed according to 3 criteria: non-response to an item greater than 5%, or item ICC less than 0.8, or variance of the item less than 1. With regards to the first criterion, some items allowed for a Not Applicable response. Items that were often not applicable were uninformative, as they did not contribute to the final score. For each item, there were 174 opportunities for a response (58 studies x 3 rounds). A 5% non-response for an item approximately equated to 9 times "NA" was answered. The 5% cut-off was chosen a priori. The item ICC is a measure of the consistency (reliability) of how an item is answered. Items that are unreliable may be thought of as being erroneous and targets for removal. Instead of using ANOVA to examine variances of MICE scores between studies and between rounds as in Table 6 and Table 8, variances of item responses were analysed for each item between rounds and between studies, i.e. items should be answered consistently from round to round (see Table 18.) The ICC applied was a 2-way random effects ICC using absolute agreement and single measures. The threshold of 0.8 was chosen a priori.

With regards to the third criterion, the variance of the item is the variance of its response. If an item is answered identically for every round and every study (has a variance of 0), it cannot discriminate between studies of different quality (125) (p. 93). A cut-off variance of 1 was chosen a priori. Table 19 shows results of item non-response, ICC and variances.

Item	Primary author	Round 1	Round 2	Round 3
...	...	...	...	...
1	Bunse	6.00	4.00	5.00
1	Canfora	5.00	6.00	5.00
1	Golden	3.00	2.00	3.00
1	Hu	3.00	6.00	4.00
...	...	...	...	...
2	Bunse	5.00	3.00	4.00
2	Canfora	4.00	4.00	4.00
2	Golden	3.00	6.00	4.00
2	Hu	5.00	5.00	5.00
...	...	...	...	...
80	Bunse	2.00	3.00	2.00
80	Canfora	3.00	4.00	3.00
80	Golden	3.00	4.00	3.00
80	Hu	1.00	3.00	2.00
...	...	...	...	...

Table 18. Example of item responses organised to allow calculation of item ICC (ANOVA compares rounds against studies per item.)

The purpose of item reduction is to improve the efficiency of a scale but not at the expense of its soundness. Loss of items necessarily reduces content validity but can also affect face, criterion and construct validity. Thus, some items that met the above criteria were kept because of their importance to validity. Such decisions were based on subjective opinion.

The questionnaire was reduced to 38 items (MICE-38), which are explained and elaborated on in detail in Chapter 4. It can be applied in 20 minutes. Because removing items affects reliability and validity measures, all tests as described for the MICE-80 questionnaire were repeated for MICE-38. Due to limitation of time, the MICE-38 version was not tested on a new set of studies. Instead, the original spreadsheet for recording item responses during the MICE-80 test-retest reliability assessment was adjusted. Items were removed, as indicated in Table 19, from the spreadsheet to produce a 38-item set of data with which to perform the tests applied to the original 80-item data. Normality tests were also repeated.

3.9. MICE-38 Reliability Tests

The 38-item data set underwent the same reliability analysis as the 80-item data, i.e. use of ANOVA and ICC (2-way random effects, absolute agreement, single measures). The results are shown in Table 20 and Table 21.

MICE-80 Item	MICE-38 Item	Non-response	Standard deviation	Variance	ICC	95% CI
01	01	0.0%	1.820	3.311	.834	.757 - .892
02		0.0%	1.453	2.111	.706	.579 - .806
03		0.0%	1.315	1.730	.701	.566 - .804
04		0.0%	1.246	1.553	.631	.497 - .746
05	02	0.0%	2.436	5.932	.975	.962 - .984
06	03	0.0%	1.855	3.441	.917	.876 - .947
07	04	0.0%	2.032	4.128	.979	.968 - .987
08		0.0%	1.006	1.012	.379	.197 - .550
09		0.0%	1.150	1.323	.597	.421 - .733
10	05	0.0%	1.899	3.606	.856	.789 - .907
11		0.0%	1.744	3.042	.704	.587 - .800
12		0.0%	0.915	0.838	.973	.959 - .983
13	06	0.0%	2.016	4.066	.918	.874 - .948
14		0.0%	1.309	1.712	.684	.468 - .814
15	07	0.0%	2.099	4.405	.882	.821 - .925
16	08	0.0%	2.500	6.250	.931	.895 - .956
17	09	0.0%	2.321	5.386	.916	.873 - .946
18	10	0.0%	2.024	4.095	.931	.895 - .956
19	11	0.0%	1.825	3.330	.906	.852 - .942
20		0.0%	1.913	3.660	.789	.669 - .870
21*	12	0.0%	0.469	0.220*	.974	.960 - .984
22*	13	0.0%	0.340	0.115*	.852	.783 - .904
23	14	0.0%	1.738	3.021	.851	.782 - .903
24		8.0%	1.230	1.514	.648	.512 - .764
25		33.9%	1.014	1.028	.355	.160 - .555
26		33.9%	1.038	1.077	.737	.598 - .842
27		0.0%	1.367	1.869	.644	.505 - .758
28		0.0%	1.532	2.348	.796	.707 - .866
29		0.0%	1.441	2.075	.708	.592 - .804
30	15	0.0%	1.679	2.818	.954	.930 - .971
31	16	0.0%	1.500	2.249	.950	.920 - .969
32	17	0.0%	1.227	1.506	.894	.843 - .932
33		0.0%	0.715	0.512	.900	.851 - .936
34	18	0.0%	2.379	5.659	.896	.846 - .934
35		16.7%	0.490	0.240	1.000	1.000 - 1.000
36		87.9%	0.218	0.048	^	
37	19	4.6%	1.164	1.355	.885	.827 - .927
38*	20	25.9%*	1.046	1.094	.865	.783 - .922
39		47.1%	1.104	1.218	.802	.666 - .896
40		90.2%	0.795	0.632	^	
41		94.3%	1.101	1.211	^	
42		87.9%	0.658	0.433	^	
43		24.1%	1.162	1.350	.966	.941 - .982
44		42.0%	0.449	0.201	.528	.323 - .710
45		0.0%	0.199	0.040	.856	.789 - .907
46*	21	0.0%	0.610	0.372*	.954	.930 - .971
47*	22	1.7%	0.746	0.556*	.979	.968 - .987
48	23	0.0%	2.425	5.879	.923	.884 - .951
49	24	0.0%	2.009	4.035	.924	.886 - .952
50	25	0.0%	2.181	4.756	.988	.982 - .993
51	26	0.0%	1.627	2.646	.860	.794 - .909

52		78.2%	1.684	2.834	.919	.799 - .975
53		37.4%	1.495	2.234	.809	.695 - .890
54		33.9%	0.968	0.936	.559	.378 - .719
55	27	0.0%	1.236	1.527	.959	.938 - .974
56		0.0%	0.379	0.144	.921	.881 - .949
57*	28	0.0%	0.772	0.596*	1.000	1.000 - 1.000
58		0.0%	1.583	2.505	.645	.513 - .757
59	29	0.0%	1.175	1.382	.856	.788 - .907
60	30	0.0%	1.430	2.046	.816	.734 - .880
61*	31	0.0%	0.491	0.241*	.811	.724 - .877
62		0.0%	0.131	0.017	1.000	1.000 - 1.000
63*	32	0.0%	0.462	0.213*	.920	.880 - .949
64*	33	0.0%	0.483	0.233*	.878	.819 - .921
65		0.0%	0.183	0.033	1.000	1.000 - 1.000
66		0.0%	0.810	0.656	.991	.987 - .995
67	34	0.0%	1.668	2.782	.853	.784 - .904
68	35	0.0%	1.698	2.884	.923	.884 - .951
69	36	0.0%	1.773	3.143	.810	.725 - .875
70	37	0.0%	2.223	4.941	.884	.827 - .925
71		0.0%	1.373	1.884	.613	.476 - .732
72		24.7%	1.841	3.388	.833	.735 - .903
73	38	0.0%	1.893	3.585	.864	.793 - .914
74		0.0%	0.540	0.292	.922	.883 - .950
75		0.0%	1.259	1.586	.741	.634 - .827
76		0.0%	0.910	0.828	.973	.958 - .983
77		0.0%	1.452	2.107	.610	.471 - .731
78		0.0%	1.253	1.569	.691	.570 - .791
79		0.0%	0.487	0.237	.952	.927 - .970
80		0.0%	1.284	1.648	.719	.595 - .815

Table 19. Item non-response, ICC and variance.

Bold face indicates items removed and the criteria for removal. An * indicates items retained despite meeting criteria. A ^ indicates inability of SPSS to calculate an ICC because one or more rounds had zero variance. Refer to Appendix B for dropped item questions.

The effect of removing more than half the items from the MICE-80 questionnaire reduced study scores by only an average of 0.054 points (standard deviation = 0.051, p = 0.000) as shown by paired samples t-test in Table 22 and Wilcoxon signed rank test in Table 23. The small change in score in relation to the large removal of items was encouraging because item reduction should not interfere with a scale's ability to measure its construct. In other words, if removing many items had greatly changed scores of the same studies, then the question arises whether the construct under measure is still the same or if another construct is being tapped. Mathematically the small difference observed can be explained, since the non-response and item variance criteria removed items that did not tend to differentiate studies.

Primary author	Round 1	Δ	Round 2	Δ	Round 3	Δ	Mean Δ
Computer science							
Ali Babar (187)	.563	-.037	.625	-.022	.608	-.023	-.027
Ali Babar (188)	.603	-.032	.609	-.060	.592	-.056	-.049
Anda (189)	.466	-.058	.443	-.080	.443	-.072	-.070
Arisholm (190)	.545	.041	.528	.033	.528	.027	.034
Briand (157)	.520	-.079	.603	-.039	.581	-.038	-.052
Bunse (191)	.564	-.032	.609	-.036	.589	-.053	-.041
Canfora (192)	.631	.028	.620	-.018	.626	-.000	.003
Golden (193)	.432	-.082	.426	-.120	.426	-.109	-.104
Hu (194)	.352	-.037	.369	-.066	.341	-.066	-.056
Johnson (195)	.508	-.074	.492	-.082	.486	-.099	-.085
Lopes (196)	.295	-.121	.330	-.125	.318	-.130	-.125
Lott (197)	.598	-.013	.581	-.018	.581	-.016	-.016
Muller (198)	.531	-.015	.587	-.012	.559	-.006	-.011
Myers (199)	.441	-.069	.452	-.100	.424	-.104	-.091
Myrtveit (156)	.472	.021	.514	-.031	.492	-.027	-.012
Ng (200)	.500	-.021	.478	-.043	.483	-.028	-.031
Prechelt (201)	.461	-.020	.489	-.021	.467	-.017	-.019
Prechelt (202)	.486	.023	.511	-.009	.506	-.000	.004
Prechelt (203)	.536	-.004	.508	-.026	.520	-.017	-.015
Prechelt (204)	.511	-.008	.533	-.021	.528	-.015	-.015
Sears (205)	.506	.013	.533	-.015	.528	-.006	-.003
Sonnenwald (206)	.661	-.035	.706	-.024	.700	-.017	-.025
Vokac (207)	.616	.052	.594	.041	.599	.055	.049
Wojcicki (208)	.463	-.054	.469	-.082	.475	-.064	-.067
Zettel (209)	.600	-.002	.589	-.008	.600	.001	-.003
Health informatics							
Bonevski (212)	.619	-.015	.597	-.032	.614	-.029	-.025
Brownbridge (213)	.313	-.125	.262	-.135	.330	-.107	-.122
Cannon (214)	.453	-.138	.346	-.152	.358	-.150	-.147
Christakis (215)	.609	-.054	.659	-.033	.637	-.046	-.044
Demakis (216)	.654	.010	.620	-.026	.626	-.012	-.010
Dexter (217)	.575	-.023	.542	-.059	.536	-.053	-.045
Fitzmaurice (218)	.346	-.023	.318	-.044	.341	-.042	-.036
Fitzmaurice (219)	.536	-.080	.494	-.080	.511	-.063	-.074
Gonzalez (220)	.514	-.056	.486	-.107	.497	-.078	-.081
Hickling (221)	.469	-.111	.408	-.163	.425	-.140	-.138
Horn (222)	.268	-.120	.257	-.128	.240	-.166	-.138
Kuperman (223)	.380	-.198	.324	-.211	.335	-.206	-.205
Lewis (224)	.542	.005	.514	-.067	.506	-.088	-.050
Lowensteyn (225)	.580	.032	.602	-.002	.602	-.006	.008
Mazzuca (226)	.564	-.021	.631	-.063	.615	-.053	-.046
McAlister (227)	.648	-.031	.693	-.030	.653	-.038	-.033
McDonald (228)	.436	-.070	.570	-.080	.536	-.075	-.075
Poller (229)	.559	-.040	.564	-.056	.581	-.052	-.049
Rosser (230)	.443	-.072	.528	-.083	.523	-.077	-.077
Rossi (231)	.727	-.027	.699	-.046	.653	-.051	-.042
Rotman (232)	.615	-.086	.665	-.074	.654	-.075	-.078
Ryff-de Leche (233)	.458	-.082	.419	-.099	.464	-.086	-.089
Schriger (234)	.778	-.005	.784	-.019	.790	-.019	-.014
Selker (235)	.799	.027	.810	.048	.810	.033	.036
Tamblyn (236)	.749	-.022	.778	.013	.754	.011	.001
Tang (237)	.380	-.096	.425	-.125	.402	-.123	-.115
Thomas (238)	.413	-.085	.374	-.130	.391	-.117	-.111

Tierney (239)	.514	-.091	.531	-.078	.508	-.094	-.088
Vadher (240)	.709	-.006	.687	-.012	.704	-.002	-.007
Vadher (241)	.436	-.098	.531	-.044	.503	-.056	-.066
Verner (242)	.402	-.137	.402	-.143	.419	-.139	-.140
Wexler (243)	.274	-.072	.318	-.101	.313	-.091	-.088
Young (244)	.244	-.092	.290	-.120	.278	-.129	-.114

Table 20. Final scores for studies recalculated with the 38-item data set.

Δ: change from 80-item data set.

	Round 1	Round 2	Round 3
N	58	58	58
Mean	.515	.523	.519
Median	.514	.530	.521
Standard deviation	.125	.131	.126
Variance	.016	.017	.016
Skewness	-.002	-.071	-.024
Standard error of skewness	.314	.314	.314
Kurtosis	-.039	-.351	-.175
Standard error of kurtosis	.618	.618	.618

Table 21. Summary statistics for final scores recalculated using the 38-item data set.

Data set	N^	Mean MICE score	Standard deviation
80-item	58	.573	.096
38-item	58	.519	.126
Mean difference .054 (95% CI .040 - .067)			
Standard deviation .051			
t 8.031			
df 57			
p (2-tailed) .000			

Table 22. Paired samples t-test between mean scores of 80 and 38-item data sets.

^: scores averaged over 3 rounds therefore N = 58.

	N^	Mean rank	Sum of ranks
Negative ranks (38-item < 80-item)	51	31.78	1621.00
Positive ranks (38-item > 80-item)	7	12.86	90.00
Ties (38-item = 80-item)	0		
Z −5.927			
p (2-tailed) .000			

Table 23. Wilcoxon signed rank test between mean scores of 80 and 38-item data sets.

^: scores averaged over 3 rounds therefore N = 58.

Most notably, as shown in Table 24, the ICC remained high after item reduction (0.963, 95% CI 0.944 - 0.977). The MICE-38 ICC improved slightly and was narrower in its confidence interval compared to the MICE-80 ICC (0.935, 95% CI 0.884 - 0.962). This is the effect of the second reduction criterion, which removed less consistent items.

		Sum of squares	df	Mean square	F	p
Between Studies		2.704	57	.047		
Within Studies	Between Rounds	.002	2	.001	1.549	.217
	Residual	.067	114	.001		
	Total	.069	116	.001		
Total		2.772	173	.016		
ICC .963 (95% CI .944 - .977)						

Table 24. ANOVA and ICC results for 38-item data set (MICE-38).

3.10. MICE-38 Normality Tests

Normality tests were performed as for the 80-item data set on the 38-item data set. Examining all scores, skewness and kurtosis were again near zero (see Table 21), and the ratios to their standard errors were between −2 and 2. Histograms of individual rounds/all scores and the Q-Q plot of all scores also supported near normality (Figure 13, Figure 14). The Shapiro-Wilks test on scores from

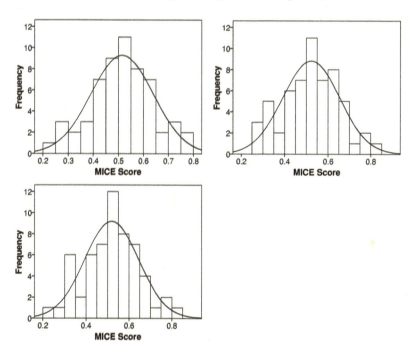

Figure 13. Histogram of MICE scores for the 38-item data set for round 1 (top left), 2 (top right) and 3 of test-retest reliability assessment.

85

all rounds was not significant (Shapiro-Wilks statistic = 0.988, df = 174, p = 0.139), again indicating normality.

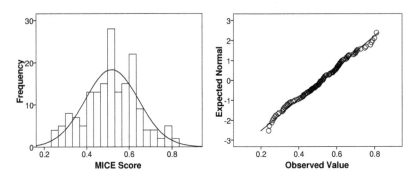

Figure 14. Histogram (left) and Q-Q plot of MICE scores for the 38-item data set (from all rounds of test-retest reliability assessment).

For the samples involved in convergent construct validity testing (statistician assistance), statistics and plots again showed near normal distributions (see Table 25, Figure 15, Figure 16, Figure 17 and Figure 18.)

	Statistician-assisted sample	Statistician-unassisted sample
Including item		
Skewness (SE)	-.658 (.536)	.047 (.374)
Kurtosis (SE)	1.333 (1.038)	.442 (.733)
Shapiro-Wilks statistic	.969	.970
Shapiro-Wilks df	18	40
Shapiro-Wilks p	.788	.369
Excluding item		
Skewness (SE)	-.658 (.536)	.049 (.374)
Kurtosis (SE)	1.333 (1.038)	.443 (.733)
Shapiro-Wilks statistic	.969	.970
Shapiro-Wilks df	18	40
Shapiro-Wilks p	.788	.368

Table 25. Normality statistics for samples used in MICE-38 convergent construct validity tests (samples with and without statistical assistance).

SE: standard error.

For known-groups testing (dichotomisation by McMaster score), the high quality sample was approximately normal (Table 26, Figure 19). However, the low quality sample was skewed to the

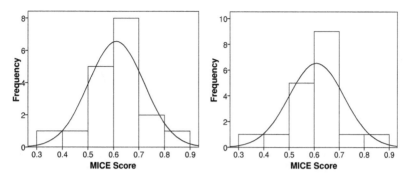

Figure 15. Histogram of MICE-38 scores for the statistician-assisted sample including (left) and excluding the item inquiring about assistance (see p. 76.)

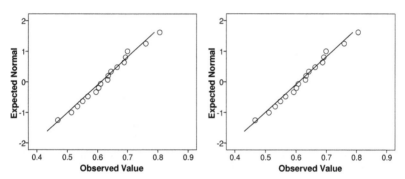

Figure 16. Normal Q-Q plots of MICE-38 scores for the statistician-assisted sample including (left) and excluding the item inquiring about assistance (see p. 76.)

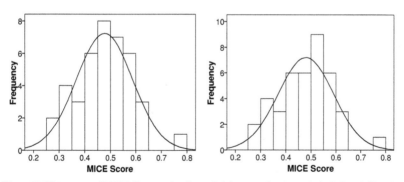

Figure 17. Histograms of MICE-38 scores for the statistician-unassisted sample including (left) and excluding the item inquiring about assistance (see p. 76.)

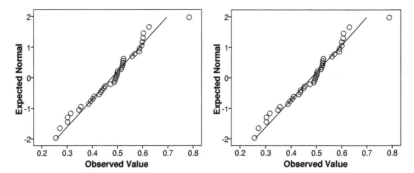

Figure 18. Normal Q-Q plots of MICE-38 scores for the statistician-unassisted sample including (left) and excluding the item inquiring about assistance (see p. 76.)

right due to an outlier (Table 26, Figure 20). It was not strongly skewed, but this sample was small (N = 10). A t-test was performed but should be interpreted with care. In this case, there is a stronger argument for use of nonparametric tests (245) (p. 465).

	McMaster score <6	McMaster score >=6
Skewness (SE)	1.689 (.687)*	-.184 (.481)
Kurtosis (SE)	3.555 (1.334)*	.466 (.935)
Shapiro-Wilks statistic	.835	.973
Shapiro-Wilks df	10	23
Shapiro-Wilks p	.039*	.762

Table 26. Normality statistics for samples used in MICE-38 known-groups criterion validity tests (dichotomised into samples of high and low quality studies).

*: non-normality; SE: standard error.

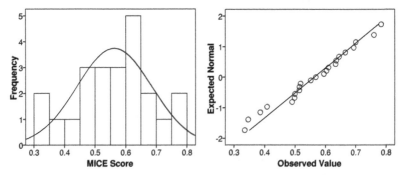

Figure 19. Histogram (left) and normal Q-Q plot of MICE-38 scores dichotomised according the McMaster scale as high quality studies (score >=6) (see p. 74.)

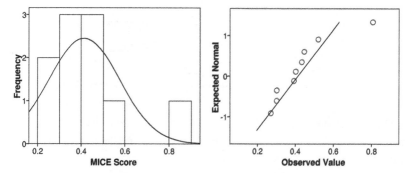

Figure 20. Histogram (left) and normal Q-Q plot of MICE-38 scores dichotomised according the McMaster scale as low quality studies (score <6) (see p. 74.)

3.11. MICE-38 Validity Tests

The same tests that were applied to the 80-item data set were applied to the 38-item data set (known-groups approach using the Garg et al review paper, JIF as a criterion standard, statistician assistance for convergent construct validity and report variables for divergent construct validity). The same parametric and nonparametric tests were applied. Appendix C contains the raw data. Face and content validity were assumed since a large number of items remained.

The MICE-38 questionnaire maintained known-groups validity. Table 27, Table 28 and Table 29 show statistically significant difference between poor and good studies. As with the 80-item results, good studies produced a higher MICE score than poor ones, though the difference between groups was slightly broader with the 38-item questionnaire. Levene's test was not significant (p = 0.703), but this did not affect t-test significance. Wilcoxon rank sum test also supported that the 38-item questionnaire could differentiate groups (p = 0.008).

McMaster score	N	Mean MICE score	Standard deviation
>=6 (good quality)	23	.563	.123
<6 (poor quality)	10	.413	.163

Table 27. Descriptive statistics of MICE scores from the 38-item data set dichotomised into good and poor quality group studies.

	Levene's test		t-test (2-tailed)			
	F	p	t	df	p	Mean difference (95% CI)
Equal variances assumed	.148	.703	2.920	31	.006	.150 (.045 - .254)
Equal variances not assumed			2.608	13.649	.021	.150 (.026 - .273)

Table 28. 2-tailed independent samples t-test comparing the means of MICE scores from good and poor quality groups, using the 38-item data set.

89

McMaster score	N	Mean rank	Sum of ranks
>=6 (good quality)	23	19.96	459.00
<6 (poor quality)	10	10.20	102.00
Wilcoxon W 102.00 p (2-tailed) .008			

Table 29. Wilcoxon rank sum test comparing MICE scores from good and poor quality groups, using the 38-item data set.

Regarding the usefulness of the JIF as a criterion standard, the correlation between JIF and MICE scores for the 38-item data set was again weak (Pearson r = 0.271, 2-tailed p = 0.079; Spearman rho = 0.297, 2-tailed p = 0.053). Figure 21 shows the scatterplot.

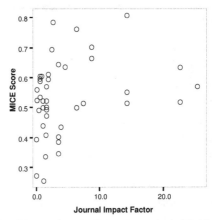

Figure 21. Scatterplot of MICE scores from the 38-item data set vs. studies' Journal Impact Factor.

The convergent construct validity hypothesis was reaffirmed with the 38-item data set (Table 30, Table 31, Table 32). The improvement in MICE score with statistical assistance was greater than seen with the 80-item questionnaire (0.129 points vs. 0.097). As before, the results are shown for the inclusion and exclusion of the statistical assistance item, which did not make a large difference.

	Statistician	N	Mean MICE score	Standard deviation
Item included	Yes	18	.611	.109
	No	40	.477	.110
Item excluded	Yes	18	.609	.110
	No	40	.480	.111

Table 30. Descriptive statistics of MICE scores from the 38-item data set for studies where statistical assistance was and was not provided.

See p. 76 for explanation of item exclusion.

90

		Levene's test		t-test (2-tailed)			
		F	p	t	df	p	Mean difference (95% CI)
Item included	Equal variances assumed	.071	.791	4.291	56	.000	.134 (.071 - .197)
	Equal variances not assumed			4.304	33.076	.000	.134 (.071 - .197)
Item excluded	Equal variances assumed	.073	.788	4.116	56	.000	.129 (.066 - .192)
	Equal variances not assumed			4.128	33.071	.000	.129 (.066 - .193)

Table 31. 2-tailed independent samples t-test comparing the means of MICE scores from studies that had and did not have statistician assistance, using the 38-item data set.

See p. 76 for explanation of item exclusion.

	Statistician	N	Mean rank	Sum of ranks
Item included	Yes	18	42.75	769.50
	No	40	23.54	941.50
	Wilcoxon W 941.50 p (2-tailed) .000			
Item excluded	Yes	18	42.61	767.00
	No	40	23.60	944.00
	Wilcoxon W 944.00 p (2-tailed) .000			

Table 32. Wilcoxon rank sum test comparing MICE scores of studies that had and did not have statistician assistance, using the 38-item data set.

See p. 76 for explanation of item exclusion.

Divergent construct validity tests for the 38-item questionnaire again showed that variables hypothetically unrelated to experimental quality exhibited low correlations (see Table 33 and Figure 22.)

	N	Author	p	Page	p	Reference	p	Year	p
r	58	.118	.377	-.054	.689	.165	.217	-.019	.888
rho	58	.108	.420	-.038	.774	.149	.265	.044	.742

Table 33. Pearson and Spearman correlation between 38-item data set MICE scores and counts of authors, pages and references and year of publication.

In summary, the reduction of the 80-item questionnaire (MICE-80) to 38 items (MICE-38) did not adversely affect criterion and construct validity. Indeed, known-groups and convergent construct validity tests demonstrated more marked results with MICE-38 and thus supported validity greater than with MICE-80.

3.12. Discussion

This chapter described the development processes used to create the MICE index, the tests used to establish reliability and validity and the results of those tests. A large literature survey was performed in the disciplines of computer science, health informatics and medicine. No completely

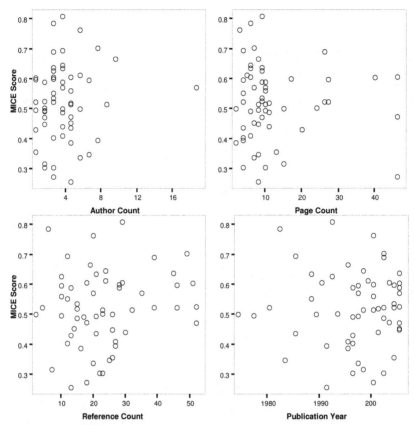

Figure 22. Scatterplots of MICE scores from the 38-item data set vs. studies' number of authors, pages, references and publication year.

adequate scales could be found in the informatics space. Existing informatics scales had questionable reliability, and none were validity tested. MICE questionnaire items were derived from a large pool of experimental concepts from a large number of publications. In addition, expert opinion contributed. Both the 80-item and the 38-item questionnaires were shown to be highly reliable using the test-retest method and intraclass correlation coefficients. Face validity and content validity were not formally tested, but it was assumed that these had been satisfied. Both questionnaires demonstrated convergent construct validity; it was hypothesised in advance that the assistance of a statistical expert in the conduct of experiments should lead to higher MICE scores. This was shown to be the case. Both questionnaires also exhibited divergent construct validity;

report variables (number of authors, pages, references and publication year) that should not be related to experimental quality were shown to have low correlations with MICE scores.

Hence, the 3 hypotheses of this research were demonstrated. With regards to the first hypothesis (p. 26), the MICE index is a questionnaire instrument that usefully measures informatics experimental quality involving human participants. With regards to the second and third hypotheses, it is applicable to computer science and health informatics domains.

The testing stages were not only beneficial in establishing the MICE index's psychometric properties but also created new information useful to research methodology. Because psychometric evaluation of controlled experimental quality in informatics is young, there are no gold criterion standards against which to assess new scales. MICE's validity tests examined whether Journal Impact Factor could be useful as a criterion standard. Unfortunately, JIF was weakly correlated with the MICE scores for both questionnaires. Nevertheless, such information creates and adds to a body of empirical evidence. No other researchers have attempted to correlate JIF to informatics experimental quality.

One of the important contributions of the MICE index is as a criterion standard. A major problem of other informatics experimental quality scales is that none had tested validity. Reasons could include lack of criterion standards, the effort involved (138) (p. 132), the uncertainty of how to proceed and being satisfied with face validity. The MICE index could be used to test other informatics experimental quality scales developed in the future.

Further new and useful information was discovered during the testing stages. MICE scores were empirically found to be near-normally distributed. No such evidence has been reported in the informatics literature before. Therefore, this research will help to establish whether normality constraints can be assumed for statistical analyses of experimental quality.

Chapter 4: The MICE Index and its Explanation

4.1.   Introduction

This chapter is the realisation of this research: a useful questionnaire instrument for measuring the quality of controlled experiments with human participants in computer science and health informatics.

The previous chapter dealt with the creation and testing process of the MICE index according to psychometric theory. Both the MICE-80 and MICE-38 questionnaires were demonstrated to be reliable and valid. Because MICE-38 is as useful as MICE-80 and is shorter, MICE-38 is the preferred version of the index. Items that were removed can be found in Appendix B. This chapter presents the 38-item questionnaire. Each item's meaning and importance to experimental quality is described; the MICE index looks for internal and external validity and whether an experimental report accurately and clearly conveys experimental conduct and results. Explanations are presented in the manner of previous experimental guidelines (see (122) and (108).)

In the questionnaire, some item questions are followed by *italicised* text, which provides further elaboration and/or instructions on how to answer. Items are organised to similarly follow the section organisations commonly found in experimental reports: introduction, method, results and discussion.

4.2.   MICE-38 Questionnaire

INSTRUCTIONS TO USERS

The Measurement of Informatics Controlled Experiments (MICE) index is a measurement tool to assess the quality of controlled experiments performed in informatics. It is used for experiments where humans receive informational support from informatics artefacts, e.g. information technologies and paper-based algorithms. It can also be used in experiments assessing the methods by which humans develop information technologies (e.g. software and interface development). It can be applied to summative or formative experiments. Users of this index should be knowledgeable in experimental design, statistical analysis and informatics. To calculate the index's score, sum the responses of each item and divide by the total possible score (the sum of maximum responses of applicable items). For items 19 and 20, "If applicable" means, "If the study design is at risk of the effect." If applicable, determine the degree of control. If the study design is not at risk, then answer as "NA". The MICE index should be applied to a single report, i.e. not to an experiment published over several reports; the score is for a single report.

INTRODUCTION
1. How clear is the rationale for the experiment? *Why was conducting the experiment important? What is the deficiency in knowledge that the experiment tried to address?*
|0 unclear| |1| |2| |3 moderately clear| |4| |5| |6 clear|

METHOD - GENERAL
2. How adequately stated are the null and/or alternative hypotheses?
|0 inadequate| |1| |2| |3 moderately adequate| |4| |5| |6 adequate|

3. How adequate is the general description of the experimental design e.g. blocked, nested, crossed, crossover, parallel group, balanced?
|0 inadequate| |1| |2| |3 moderately adequate| |4| |5| |6 adequate|

4. Is the experimental design suitable for the experimental questions posed?
|0 unsuitable| |1| |2| |3 moderately suitable| |4| |5| |6 suitable|

METHOD - TREATMENT (INDEPENDENT VARIABLE)
5. Are the treatments suitable for the experimental questions posed?
|0 unsuitable| |1| |2| |3 moderately suitable| |4| |5| |6 suitable|

METHOD - SETTING
6. Is the site representative of a real-world setting in which the technology/method would be used? *If the site is not described then answer "NA".*
|0 not representative| |1| |2| |3 moderately representative| |4| |5| |6 representative|
|-- NA|

METHOD - EXPERIMENTAL UNIT (PARTICIPANTS)
7. Is it clear how the experimental units were sampled e.g. random, pseudorandom, convenience?
|0 unclear| |1| |2| |3 moderately clear| |4| |5| |6 clear|

8. Are inclusion criteria for the experimental unit clear?
|0 unclear| |1| |2| |3 moderately clear| |4| |5| |6 clear|

9. Are exclusion criteria for the experimental unit clear?
|0 unclear| |1| |2| |3 moderately clear| |4| |5| |6 clear|

10. Is the experimental unit level, e.g. individual, group, organisation, suitable for the experimental questions posed?
|0 unsuitable| |1| |2| |3 moderately suitable| |4| |5| |6 suitable|

11. How representative are the experimental units of the real world? *If the experimental unit is unclear then answer "NA".*
|0 not representative| |1| |2| |3 moderately representative| |4| |5| |6 representative|
|-- NA|

METHOD - ALLOCATION/RANDOMISATION
12. Was the allocation completely random? *Merely stating random is insufficient – the technique is required e.g. computer-generated.*
|0 no or unknown| |1 yes|

13. Did investigators use allocation concealment techniques e.g. central randomising agent, sequentially numbered opaque envelopes, randomising at time of allocation? *Allocation concealment requires that the investigators could not have subverted (random) allocation by knowing ahead of the time of allocation to which group a participant would go.*
|0 no or unknown| |1 yes|

METHOD - MATERIALS
14. Is it clear what the supporting experimental materials are i.e. hardware, tools, software, documentation, or other supporting items? *This does not refer to measurement instrumentation for the experiment.*
|0 unclear| |1| |2| |3 moderately clear| |4| |5| |6 clear|

METHOD - OUTCOMES (DEPENDENT VARIABLES)
15. Are the measurement methods, instruments or outcomes reliable? *Reliability is the consistency of a measure. Are reliability coefficients stated? Have instruments been previously shown to be reliable?*
|0 unknown| |1 overall poorly reliable| |2| |3 overall moderately reliable| |4| |5|
      |6 overall highly reliable|

16. Are the measurement methods, instruments or outcomes valid? *Validity is whether observations actually do measure what they intended to measure. Are measures face valid, criterion valid, construct valid etc?*
|0 unknown| |1 overall poorly valid| |2| |3 overall moderately valid| |4| |5| |6 overall highly valid|

17. What percentage of main/primary outcomes are objective e.g. not subject to interpretation, recall error etc?
|0 0%-25%| |1 26%-50%| |2 51%-75%| |3 76%-100%|

METHOD - BIAS/CONFOUNDING
18. Are the control and treatment groups comparable in important ways (apart from the independent variables)? *If insufficient information then answer "Not comparable".*
|0 not comparable, confounding highly likely| |1| |2| |3 moderately comparable, confounding moderately likely| |4| |5| |6 comparable, confounding unlikely|

19. If applicable, do the investigators control for the learning effect e.g. training sessions, analysis of treatment sequence? *Treatment can be confounded with subject familiarity (becoming more familiar) with the technology/method or task. Within-subject designs are at risk.*
|0 not controlled or acknowledged| |1inadequate control| |2 controlled but effect not quantified|
      |3 effect quantified| |-- NA|

20. If applicable, do the investigators control for carryover or contamination effects? *The effect of a treatment can persist (carry over) into the control state e.g. a crossover design, or affect the control group as well as the treatment group (contamination).*
|0 not controlled or acknowledged| |1inadequate control| |2 controlled but effect not quantified|
      |3 effect quantified| |-- NA|

21. Are relevant subjects blind to expectation effects e.g. blind to treatment group, blind to experimental hypothesis? *Proponents and critics of technologies and methods may be biased due to expectation effects, which can affect self-reported and/or performance outcomes. Relevant subjects are those whose observations may be influenced by expectation effect.*
|0 no or unknown| |1 partially| |2 yes|

22. Are assessors of outcomes blind to expectation effects e.g. blind to treatment group, hypothesis? *If all outcomes are self-reported then answer "NA".*
|0 no or unknown| |1 partially| |2 yes| |-- NA|

RESULTS - GENERAL

23. How adequate is the baseline comparison of the characteristics of experimental groups? *Is there enough information to tell whether groups were comparable or not?*
|0 inadequate| |1| |2| |3 moderately adequate| |4| |5| |6 adequate|

24. How adequately are effect sizes presented?
|0 inadequate| |1| |2| |3 moderately adequate| |4| |5| |6 adequate|

25. To what extent are confidence intervals used?
|0 not used| |1| |2| |3 moderately used| |4| |5| |6 widely used|

RESULTS - INELIGIBLE/LOST DATA

26. Is it clear how many participants were eligible, were enrolled, and were lost, excluded or had withdrawn?
|0 unclear| |1| |2| |3 moderately clear| |4| |5| |6 clear|

27. What is the percentage of lost/withdrawn/excluded participants to the enrolled?
|0 unclear| |1 >20%| |2 10%-20%| |3 <10%|

RESULTS - STATISTICAL METHODS

28. Are sample sizes calculated for all main outcomes?
|0 no| |1 partially| |2 yes|

29. How appropriate is the use of scale type (level of measurement) e.g. nominal, ordinal, interval, ratio?
|0 inappropriate||1| |2| |3 moderately appropriate| |4| |5| |6 appropriate|

30. How adequate is the description of the statistical tests used e.g. name, significance level and corrections?
|0 inadequate| |1| |2| |3 moderately adequate| |4| |5| |6 adequate|

31. Are statistical test assumptions unacceptably violated? *If violations are minor or absent then answer "No".*
|0 yes| |1 no|

32. Is unit of analysis error present (and not corrected for)? *This occurs when observations are analysed without consideration of their independence e.g. analysing individual data rather than as a group (cluster) when measurements on individuals within a group would likely be similar than between groups. If corrected then answer "No".*
|0 yes| |1 no|

33. Was a statistician consulted?
|0 no or unknown| |1 yes|

34. How appropriate overall is the statistical analysis?
|0 inappropriate||1| |2| |3 moderately appropriate| |4| |5| |6 appropriate|

DISCUSSION

35. To what extent are the investigators' conclusions justified?
|0 not justified| |1| |2| |3 moderately justified| |4| |5| |6 justified|

36. How adequate is the discussion on how the findings relate to current evidence and/or theory?
|0 inadequate| |1| |2| |3 moderately adequate| |4| |5| |6 adequate|

37. How adequate is the discussion on external validity i.e. how the findings can be generalised?
|0 inadequate| |1| |2| |3 moderately adequate| |4| |5| |6 adequate|

38. How adequately do the investigators discuss the limitations of the experiment?
|0 inadequate| |1| |2| |3 moderately adequate| |4| |5| |6 adequate|

4.3. Explanation and Elaboration

4.3.1. How clear is the rationale for the experiment?

The rationale for an experiment is its raison d'être. Because controlled experiments with human participants are usually costly in time, effort and manpower, there should be good reasons to conduct them. The purpose of any empirical investigation is to determine new knowledge or provide further evidence for or against what is already suspected. Therefore, there is little point in conducting expensive experiments if they do not contribute to the knowledge base. Indeed, for medical experiments involving human participants, there is an ethical requirement from the Helsinki Declaration that such research "must be based on a thorough knowledge of the scientific literature." (252) This could potentially apply to health informatics experiments.

From a quality perspective, as defined for the MICE index, explanation of how the experiment contributes to knowledge improves understanding of the experiment. It puts into perspective the results of an experiment. It also helps external validity by assisting readers to compare the results against other studies and decide whether they can be generalised to those. Describing the rationale also alerts readers to shallow hypotheses. These are simplistic research questions that do not "reflect an underlying, explanatory theory" (122) for important phenomena in informatics.

When answering item 1, users should look for information, usually in the report's introduction, that compares the presented research against current knowledge. This item is not inquiring about the worthiness of the research problem. For example, a good research hypothesis is: medical errors are costly and could be reduced using a clinical decision support system; item 1 would be answered according to whether the experiment contributes to the evidence base that clinical decision support systems reduce medical errors and not according to the description of how much of a problem medical errors are.

4.3.2. How adequately stated are the null and/or alternative hypotheses?

Study reports usually describe the objectives, aims or goals of the experiment. This establishes whether the actual conduct of the experiment was suited to achieving the stated goals. If the design of a study is not suited to its objectives, it will have poor internal validity. Stating objectives also helps understanding by concisely describing the purpose of the experiment and by allowing readers to gauge whether the experiment is similar to others and their objectives.

In addition, by stating hypotheses formally, it forces investigators to explicitly indicate the primary outcome measures and, if any, the secondary. This alerts readers to the potential of fishing expeditions, where investigators produce spuriously statistically significant data from excessive hypotheses tests (108, 122).

The rationale for requiring null or alternative hypotheses over general statements of objectives is that the former are concise and exact ways of expressing the goals of experiments. They are also easier to find in a report, which is particularly useful when comparing findings in the results section to the original goals.

When answering item 2, users should look for null or alternative hypotheses statements, ideally indicated by H_0 or H_1/H_A. Statements should be clear and concise.

4.3.3. How adequate is the general description of the experimental design e.g. blocked, nested, crossed, crossover, parallel group, balanced?

The description of the basic design of an experiment helps to convey to the reader an overall picture of its conduct. Keywords, as mentioned in the item stem, provide concise and clear meaning. This contributes to the overall understanding of the report, in particular when the fine details of the experimental method are then explained. A general description is also helpful in quickly determining whether a chosen design is suitable for the research hypotheses. In particular it can affect the choice of statistical tests (168).

When answering item 3, users should look for a statement, ideally at the beginning of the methods section, which describes clearly and accurately the general type of experimental design used. Study design keywords are most helpful.

4.3.4. Is the experimental design suitable for the experimental questions posed?

This item is aimed at a high level of abstraction and requires a broad consideration by MICE index users. There may be many reasons why a particular experimental design is poorly suited to the research hypothesis. It is an important consideration since a poorly chosen design will adversely affect internal validity; results will often have systematic error (bias) or confounding effects. An example of poor design choice is the use of historical controls when it would be clear that secular trends could account for results. Another example is the use of a crossover study when carryover or learning effects would corrupt the second stage.

When answering item 4, users should judge whether the chosen experimental design would have caused problems for answering the research hypothesis. If the study design is poorly described, it cannot be suitable.

4.3.5. Are the treatments suitable for the experimental questions posed?

This is another item that requires broad consideration. Treatments are the conditions placed on the experimental groups to see the effect on outcomes of interest. In controlled experimentation, by definition, the research question is answered by comparing treatment groups to control groups.

Therefore, treatments that do not adequately separate groups cannot answer the research question at hand. This also implies that treatments are well-defined. There may be more than one treatment that is recognised by the investigators. An example is the study by Fitzmaurice et al (218). The aim of the controlled trial was to determine whether International Normalized Ratio (INR) control for general practice patients improved using a decision support system for dosing warfarin. The treatment was the use of the system by general practitioners, and the control was management by hospital haematologists without the system. Hence, the additional treatment not considered by Fitzmaurice et al was management by specialist doctors, which could have accounted for differences in INR stability.

When answering item 5, users should judge whether the defined treatments would have caused problems for answering the research question. Users should consider whether treatment and control statuses adequately differentiated participants and whether all relevant treatments were addressed. Poor definitions of treatments should be considered unsuitable.

4.3.6. Is the site representative of a real-world setting in which the technology/method would be used?

A real-world setting is distinct from an artificially created environment such as a laboratory. Credible results are most useful when they are generated in a real working environment, e.g. a hospital, a clinic or industry. Such results are more likely to be externally valid and useful to readers of a report since they can compare their situation with the study.

This item is particularly important for computer science experiments where students are often used as experimental participants (91, 94), and therefore the site is usually a university. However, if the computing technology or method is intended for a student setting, then the choice of an academic site is acceptable. An example is computer-assisted education, where an experiment might test the hypothesis that learning is benefited.

When answering item 6, users should judge whether the site for the experiment is similar to the final working environment where the technology or method would be used.

4.3.7. Is it clear how the experimental units were sampled e.g. random, pseudorandom, convenience?

The selection of experimental units, e.g. human participants, departmental units, hospitals, companies, is always decided as part of an experimental plan. Rarely can a census be achieved, and investigators should communicate how the sampling was performed. How a sample is selected from a population can greatly affect the internal validity of an experiment. For instance, a voluntary response sample is more likely to be affected by bias than a simple random sample (245) (p. 219) because the former is more likely to attract supporters of technology, while the latter gives all people an equal chance to be selected. Computer science experiments are particularly at risk since convenience has been the main method of sampling (80) (usually from a captive audience: students taking the university course that the investigator teaches (94)).

When answering item 7, users should look for a description of the sampling method that would allow the user to make a judgement on sampling biases.

4.3.8. Are inclusion criteria for the experimental unit clear?
The experimental unit is the experimental object to which a treatment is assigned. It is often an individual human participant but can be clusters of individuals, e.g. a pair, a department, a medical ward team, a hospital or company. Knowing the characteristics of the experimental unit helps readers of a study to determine whether the results are applicable to their environment, i.e. external validity. Also, by defining entry criteria, participants are made more comparable on independent variables that are thought to affect outcomes (122).

In health informatics reports, occasionally there appears a description of patient characteristics when patients were not actually the experimental unit. Rather the health care provider was the experimental unit. This is a carryover from clinical trial reporting where patients (individuals or groups) are usually the unit of experimentation. In experiments where health care providers are assigned treatments, such as the use of a clinical information system, the description of inclusion criteria applies to the provider and not the providers' patients. However, patient demographics may be important if treatment and control provider groups see different patients and these differences would have an effect on outcomes.

When answering item 8, users should look for a clear description of the criteria that allowed entry of experimental units into the study.

4.3.9. Are exclusion criteria for the experimental unit clear?
This item is similar to item 8 but looks for characteristics of the experimental unit that denied entry into the study. Often investigators do not indicate exclusion criteria and assume that readers will guess that none existed. Ideally, if there was indeed nothing to exclude a participant from the study, it should be stated. This makes for certain to the reader that no exclusion criteria existed.

When answering item 9, users should look for a clear description of the criteria that denied entry of experimental units into the study.

4.3.10. Is the experimental unit level, e.g. individual, group, organisation, suitable for the experimental questions posed?

This item relates to whether the experimental unit has been chosen correctly for the research hypothesis. It is an issue of internal validity. In all experiments, investigators must decide what the level of the experimental unit should be. It is often an individual person but may be clusters of individuals. If an experimental unit is defined at the individual level when groups are more appropriate, the sample size will be inflated, and unit of analysis error can occur. The experimental unit should be chosen according to the research hypothesis (253). If the hypothesis concerns organisations, the experimental unit should not be individuals within the organisations and treatment assignment performed accordingly (122).

Health informatics studies are at particular risk of inappropriate choice of experimental unit. A common research hypothesis is whether the use of a clinical information system by health care providers improves practice and therefore improves patient illness outcomes. Investigators often then enrol patients into their study as the experimental unit while the treatment (the information system) is applied to the providers. If the unit of observation is the patient, the sample size will usually be greatly inflated since patients significantly outnumber providers. Consequently unit of analysis error occurs. Depending on the research hypothesis, it may be necessary to consider the experimental unit at a higher level, e.g. clinic, ward team or hospital.

When answering item 10, users should consider how severely the level of the experimental unit would cause unit of analysis error given the research hypothesis. This item differs from item 32, which inquires about the presence of unit of analysis error and whether statistical correction has been made. For item 10, ideally, units should have been defined appropriately at the planning stage of an experiment.

4.3.11. How representative are the experimental units of the real world?

This item relates to the external validity of the participants. Ideally participants would come from a real-world setting where the treatment would be used as this has high external validity. As mentioned above, computer science controlled experiments commonly utilise undergraduate university students as subjects. Depending on the research hypothesis, this can limit the generalisability of results to computing professionals, particularly when the outcomes relate to work performance. In contrast, health informatics experiments tend to use working professionals as opposed to health care students. However, again depending the research hypothesis, such experiments may not be widely externally valid since some studies focus on junior health care providers but try to extrapolate to professionals of higher experience. One example is the effect of a diagnostic system on the accuracy of a doctor's diagnosis. If an experiment is conducted on junior doctors, the effect may not be similar on senior ones (presuming the research hypothesis is the effect of a system on doctors in general). Focussing on junior doctors or health care students may be appropriate if the system is aimed at assisting a particular group, e.g. a hospital decision support system that junior doctors must consult and tends to be only used by them.

When answering item 11, users should judge how similar the experimental participants are to those in the real environment where the technology/method would be used.

4.3.12. Was the allocation completely random?

Randomisation is an important technique in controlled experimentation. By allocating treatment to participants in a random manner, bias and confounding are minimized. In particular, selection bias is eliminated (108), and unknown confounders are equally distributed among participants (155) (p. 188). Indeed, in medical experimentation and health informatics, it is considered a critical aspect. Sackett (254) wrote that readers of clinical journals who want to distinguish useful from useless or harmful therapies should ignore nonrandomised studies and "go onto the next article." As Sackett describes, there have been many examples of where lack of randomisation has lead to incorrect therapy. In Chapter 3, all of the medical scales and health informatics sources used to develop the MICE index refer to the importance of randomisation, as does Van der Loo's scale (150). Only De Keizer's health informatics scale does not because it is aimed at all types of evaluation designs, such as nonrandomised studies (135).

Because of the importance of randomisation to internal validity, this item marks down studies where a description of randomisation is absent, even if randomisation did occur. It is considered mandatory to report. Furthermore, it is defined as mandatory that the technique of randomisation be described. "Completely random" means that all participants have the same chance of being allocated a treatment. Some methods are referred to as random but are actually not sufficiently random. For instance, enrolling participants by day of the week is sometimes mistakenly considered to be random. It is pseudorandom because there may be systematic reasons why certain participants present themselves at certain times. True randomness, or as close as possible, is commonly achieved by computer generation or random numbers table.

When answering item 12, users should look for a description of how treatments were randomly allocated and assess whether the technique produced completely random (or as close as possible) assignment.

103

4.3.13. **Did investigators use allocation concealment techniques e.g. central randomising agent, sequentially numbered opaque envelopes, randomising at time of allocation?**

Randomisation of groups to treatment reduces bias and confounding, but its effectiveness can be reduced. If investigators are aware of whether a participant will subsequently receive a certain treatment, randomisation can be undermined, and the allocation process is longer completely random. Allocation concealment hides the knowledge of upcoming randomisation until the randomisation actually occurs. Just as randomisation is important for internal validity, so too is allocation concealment. Indeed, in clinical trials, studies without allocation concealment have been shown to overestimate the effect of thearpies by 30 - 41% (255). There are several techniques to implement allocation concealment. All aim to allocate treatment at the time a participant enters the study: a central randomising agent is an external service that performs the allocation; sequentially numbered opaque envelopes contain the allocation and must be followed in sequential order.

When answering item 13, users should look for a treatment allocation that does not allow investigators to have foreknowledge of which treatment is to be assigned to which participant.

4.3.14. **Is it clear what the supporting experimental materials are i.e. hardware, tools, software, documentation, or other supporting items?**

A description of the experimental materials assists readers in determining whether results can be generalised to their circumstances. The failure or success of computing technology and methods may also be related to the supporting materials employed. For example, a version of the VIE-PNN decision support system for improving prescribing of parenteral nutrition was unsuccessfully used by physicians due to its installation on a stand-alone PC, which was located away from where the physicians worked (222). When it was installed on the hospital intranet and served to workstations as HTML pages, usage was dramatically improved. Another example is the study of software programming where specialised training and reference manuals can affect programming performance (80). If readers of a study are to decide whether the results of an experiment apply to their situation, they need to know whether they own or have access to the same supporting items.

When answering item 14, users should look for a description of supporting artefacts needed to conduct the experiment and that might be needed in a real environment when applying the technology or method. This item does not inquire about materials for measuring outcomes, which are referred to in items 15 and 16.

4.3.15. **Are the measurement methods, instruments or outcomes reliable?**

Reliability of measurement is one of the pillars of measurement theory, as discussed in Chapter 2. If measurements are unreliable then, by definition, there is an unsatisfactory degree of associated error. High degree of error means that results cannot be trusted and are internally invalid. Because of this concept's importance to empirical studies, this item marks down unreported reliability. Ideally, there should be a quantification of reliability of measures, such as a correlation coefficient or a kappa statistic (122). Sometimes these measurement issues are addressed in separate papers and therefore "published elsewhere". Nevertheless, investigators should report enough information in the main paper to indicate the reliability of measures.

Reliability is a particularly important concept for informatics. Often human judges are required in determining outcomes, e.g. assessing the correctness of programmes when using a software development method or the appropriateness of drug prescribing when assisted by a clinical information system. Judges should be shown to be reliable before they are used in experiments, for example by demonstrating inter-rater agreement.

When answering item 15, users should look for a description and, ideally, a quantification of the reliability of measures.

4.3.16. Are the measurement methods, instruments or outcomes valid?

Validity is another pillar of measurement theory. Experimental measures should be valid. If measures are not valid, they do not reflect the construct being assessed and are instead tapping something else. Thus, results cannot be internally valid. It is a critical aspect of measurement, and unrecognised validity issues are therefore penalised by this item.

Validity is another common measurement problem in informatics. For example, concepts such as software complexity, user satisfaction, system benchmarking and IT security require careful consideration to what instruments dedicated to their measurement might actually be measuring. Is software complexity accurately measured by counting lines of code, or is it more related to logical statements or to programming comments? Is a survey on user satisfaction actually measuring that a system is free of faults, or that it meets user requirements, or that it is fast, or that the interface is intuitive, or other aspects (256)? System benchmarks can measure a wide range of constructs, from floating point operation of a CPU to volume testing of a database. Finally, the measurement of IT security is largely qualitative and subjective (257) where, "The scientific validation of measuring tools... raises many questions that have not been discussed not to mention answered." (258)

When answering item 16, users should look for a description of whether measures are valid. Many measures will often only have face validity, if described at all, which should be regarded as less convincing than objective criterion and construct validity testing.

4.3.17. What percentage of main/primary outcomes are objective e.g. not subject to interpretation, recall error etc?

Human memory and interpretation are fallible. Objective outcome measures are those that do not require a judgement by the producer of the outcome, e.g. time taken to accomplish a task, a numerical biochemical result, counting lines of code. When a human assessor is required to make an interpretation for a dependent variable, the outcome is no longer objective (171), e.g. judgement of source code correctness or appropriateness of clinical management. Subjective judgment is less preferred than objective because of the potential for less consistent measurement (153) (p. 67). In addition, subjective measurement can lead to expectation and observer biases (see items 21 and 22.)

When answering item 17, users should count the number of main or primary outcomes the investigators are examining and consider how many of those are objective.

4.3.18. Are the control and treatment groups comparable in important ways (apart from the independent variables)?

The power of controlled experiments comes from manipulation of variables of interest while maintaining other variables as constant, so that causal relationships can be assessed with confidence. When experimental groups only differ in the independent variable, this provides the strongest connection between cause and effect.

Comparability can be achieved by simple randomisation or stratifying groups on variables that are likely to affect outcomes, followed by randomisation. Use of within-subject designs is also helpful. Randomisation of small experimental samples, which often occur in computer science experiments, does not always produce unbiased allocation (122). In this case it becomes even more important that investigators demonstrate that confounding is not present. Randomisation, though, remains a powerful technique to make groups comparable, not least because it also evenly distributes unknown confounders (155) (p. 188). In addition to the description of how investigators made groups comparable, ideally they should include a table in their report that shows the similarity or otherwise of experimental groups with regards to potentially important variables (item 23).

Because of the importance of this experimental principle, inadequate reporting that fails to demonstrate how experimental groups compare is penalised by the MICE index.

When answering item 18, users should look for a description that compares experimental groups and judge whether the groups were similar in important ways other than in the variables being manipulated. Otherwise confounding factors could account for the results. If the study design is within-subject, then control and treatment groups are usually comparable. However, this may not always be true, e.g. fatigue effects on participant performance.

4.3.19. If applicable, do the investigators control for the learning effect e.g. training sessions, analysis of treatment sequence?

The learning effect is a form of bias where participants become more effective or perform better due to learning of the experimental tasks required or the computing technology/method. For instance, if a group of programmers are taught a new form of fault inspection, fault detection rates might improve with time as they become accustomed to the technique. The same applies to the use of information systems when there is a learning curve to overcome before the system can be used to its potential. Learning effect means that early experiments might produce poorer results than later experiments, which is the same as stating that later experiments may show better results than earlier ones. The importance of the direction of error depends on the perspective of the research (effect size is under or overestimated.) For example, with regards to an underestimation perspective, one of the largest randomised controlled trials to assess the effect of a paediatric decision support system on patient outcomes failed to produce significant benefits. The MARY system was a neonatal intensive care monitoring system and the object of a trial that lasted 33 months, enrolled 600 neonates, examined 10 outcomes and followed babies into early childhood (259). Because none of the outcomes were significantly improved, the investigators performed a human factors study (260), which observed that one of the important issues was the lack or shortage of system training. The benefit of MARY may have been underestimated because unit staff were not instructed on the more advanced functionalities (260). Training sessions or letting participants become used to a new treatment are ways to control for learning effect.

Within-subject studies are particularly at risk of learning effect because participants can learn the experimental tasks required of them and transfer the knowledge to subsequent stages of the experiment. Outcomes are then influenced by learning effect beyond the effect of treatment. This is an example of potential overestimation of effect size. It is a particular risk in computer science experiments because within-subject studies are common (16/25 [64% of] computer science experiments used to test the MICE index in Chapter 3 were within-subject designs compared to 2/33 [6% of] health informatics experiments.) Learning effect can be quantified in within-subject studies by statistical analysis of treatment sequence. Another technique to control for learning is to vary the order in which participants encounter treatments (159), such as a counterbalanced design (191). In parallel-group studies, learning effect of required tasks is potentially present but, since it affects all experimental groups (i.e. including controls), no bias occurs.

When answering item 19, users should judge whether learning effects are likely to be present to a degree that would affect internal validity. If in doubt, the NA response should be chosen. If an important learning effect was present but not recognised, this should be considered as not controlled.

4.3.20. If applicable, do the investigators control for carryover or contamination effects?

A carryover effect occurs in crossover/within-subject studies when the influence of a treatment persists into the control state. This is typically seen in pharmacological trials, where the effect of the drug given during the treatment stage carries over into when a patient enters the control stage because insufficient time is given for the drug to wash out from the patient (261, 262). Hence, the outcomes for the control state can appear more similar to the treatment state than are actually the case, and the effect size is reduced. Carryover effect in this book is considered distinct from learning effect (when the experimental tasks have been learnt), although the terms have been treated synonymously (122). Carryover effect is the effect of the treatment persisting and not experience with tasks.

Contamination occurs in parallel-group studies when the influence of a treatment spills over into the control group. Like carryover effect, the consequence is to increase the similarity between treatment and control groups and therefore reduce effect size. Sometimes the terms carryover and contamination are used synonymously (138) (p. 214) but, in this book, carryover specifically refers to crossover designs.

Health informatics experiments are particularly at risk of contamination. Patients are often assigned to a treatment group where attending health care providers use a decision support system, while control group patients are managed by unassisted providers. However, if a health care provider cares for patients from both groups, it is probable that he or she has learnt from the system and might apply that improved knowledge to control patients, hence contaminating the control group with the decision support system treatment. To control for the contamination effect, treatment allocation should occur at a higher level, such as providers or departments (138) (p. 214). Providers then retain the same level of knowledge and are consistent when they attend to patients. Contamination can still occur at the provider level if providers from different groups are, for some reason, required attend to the same patient.

When answering item 20, users should judge whether carryover or contamination effects were likely to be present to a degree that would affect internal validity. If in doubt, the NA response should be chosen. If an important carryover or contamination was present but not recognised, this should be considered as not controlled.

4.3.21. Are relevant subjects blind to expectation effects e.g. blind to treatment group, blind to experimental hypothesis?

Expectation about a new informatics technology or method can influence human participants. Critics may consciously or subconsciously underperform when assigned to the intervention or try harder when assigned as control. Enthusiasts are the opposite. In addition to performance, subjective measures can be influenced by expectation. In this case, it can be called the placebo effect, where subjects "report a favourable response" (155) (p. 192) to interventions due to their belief that the new innovations are superior.

To address expectation effects is to remove the expectation from participants. Since expectation is a state of mind, participants must be deceived so that such thoughts are not present. In medical experimentation, fake therapies are given that are indistinguishable from the real therapies, e.g. inert medicines that taste, smell and appear as the real ones; and incomplete therapeutic procedures that feel real without having performed the critical step. The process of confusing participants to experimental group status is called blinding. In informatics experiments, it is almost impossible to blind participants to experimental group because most interventions are plainly apparent, e.g. computer-based systems, man-machine interfaces. Indeed, because informatics deals with information, most interventions are educational or influence human information processing. Despite the difficulty of blinding in informatics experiments, it is important to attempt if possible. In medical experimentation, there is clear evidence that placebo effect inflates treatment effects (155) (p. 195). In the study by Lowenstein et al (225), the provision of computerised coronary risk profiles improved patient risk factors, but the computer-aided physician group was younger, more recently graduated and more likely to enrol their patients into the study than the unassisted control group (p < 0.05). It is possible that the younger physicians embraced the computer technology, and this accounted for some of the patient improvement.

One method to blind participants is to not inform them or only partially inform them of the research hypothesis. Participants will then be less likely to manipulate outcomes since they are unsure of what is being studied. While this is a useful technique from a scientific point of view, it may be unethical in health informatics experiments if the Helsinki declaration is adhered to, i.e. "Each potential subject must be adequately informed of the aims, methods… the anticipated benefits and potential risks of the study…" (252)

Another technique is to use electronic interfaces when the intervention is an electronic information resource (263). Such interfaces could secretly assign participants and deliver altered services accordingly. As Eldredge states, "Control groups can continue to receive access to conventional resources or services via the same electronic interface, whereas the intervention group can receive access to variants of the conventional resources or services as part of an intervention." (263)

Objective measures are useful as participants cannot alter their subjective outcomes, but they do not affect the motivation and performance of champions and critics.

When answering item 21, users should look for methods investigators used to manage participant expectation effects.

4.3.22. Are assessors of outcomes blind to expectation effects e.g. blind to treatment group, hypothesis?

The other important group to blind are the outcome assessors. This prevents observer (assessment, ascertainment) bias where enthusiastic or critical assessors alter their subjective assessment in favour of or against the new innovation. Indeed, even objective measures can be affected if assessors influence participant behaviour; Rosenthal and Rubin demonstrated that researchers alter the way they treat subjects if the researchers expect a certain outcome (264). If assessors know to which group a participant belongs, they may err on the side of "giving the benefit of the doubt" for intervention participants when uncertain of an outcome. Also, they may probe more deeply in the treatment arm and systematically provide more complete/accurate data (155) (p. 191). Observer bias is a particular problem when the developers of a technology are also the outcome assessors. They are the greatest champions of the intervention.

There is well-established empirical evidence that observer bias occurs in medical experiments, and that the effectiveness of therapies is erroneously inflated as a result (265, 266). In clinical trials, it would be regarded as suspicious if the developer of a therapy, e.g. a pharmaceutical company, were the sole research group to conduct an assessment of therapeutic efficacy. Indeed, such practice would have significant conflict of interest (267). Yet, the majority of controlled experiments in health informatics are performed (solely) by the developer of the technology. 20/33 (61%) health informatics studies used to test MICE's reliability (see Chapter 3) were experiments of the developers' own systems. In only 5/33 (15%) studies were the investigators clearly independent of the technology (the remaining 8 were unclear.)

Informatics is at great risk of assessment bias for also another reason. Inherently, many outcomes are based on judges' opinion. Objective measures are more resilient to observer bias than subjective. For example, in health informatics, mortality rates and biochemical markers are less susceptible to manipulation than appropriateness of therapy or disease severity.

When both experimental subjects and outcomes assessors are blinded to group assignment, this is called double blinding. While it is difficult to achieve double blinding in informatics experiments, it should be remembered that in medical experimentation, the absence of double blinding leads to more favourable outcomes for new interventions (174).

This item does not refer to blinding of the statistician (the MICE-80 questionnaire contains such an item but was removed for MICE-38.)

When answering item 22, users should look for methods investigators used to blind outcome assessors. In the case that all outcomes are self-reported by participants, then expectation (placebo) effect is potentially present rather than observation bias. In this book, observation bias is defined as the effect of external assessors, though others have considered personal observation (subjective observation) included under this concept (108).

4.3.23. How adequate is the baseline comparison of the characteristics of experimental groups?

As discussed in item 18, experimental groups should ideally be different in only the independent variable. Investigators should show that other variables that may influence outcomes have been distributed evenly between experimental groups. This is important because randomisation does not guarantee that groups will be similar in respects other than the independent variable, particularly if sample sizes are small.

When answering item 23, users should look for a clear description of the comparability of experimental groups. The most easily understood format of demonstrating comparability is to use a table. This item differs from item 18; item 18 calls for a judgement by MICE index users as to the possibility of confounding. Item 23 is related to reporting and improving the understanding of a study. If groups were not comparable, but this was reported clearly, for example in a table, item 23 can still be marked highly.

4.3.24. How adequately are effect sizes presented?

An effect size is taken by the MICE index to mean the magnitude of the treatment effect. This can standardised, e.g. Cohen's d, or unstandardised, e.g. simple raw difference between means, depending on what is most easily understood and appropriate for the outcomes measured (268). A statement about effect size is useful to readers as it conveys deliberately what the benefit of the treatment is. This is the very point of experimentation: to express how much a new informatics object or method is better or worse than its competitor, which is usually the current standard.

When answering item 24, users should judge whether the description of effect size shows how much improvement (or worsening) of outcomes the treatment caused and whether it is expressed in a form most appropriate and understood.

4.3.25. To what extent are confidence intervals used?

Data from samples represent estimates of population parameters. Therefore, confidence intervals are important to demonstrate the error associated with measurement. They also help readers of studies in the interpretation of sample size, power and statistical significance. Narrower confidence intervals indicate a more stable estimate of effect and vice versa, which is especially useful when interpreting nonsignificant results (155) (p. 253), (108). Confidence intervals can also provide the same information as p values in terms of statistical significance (155) (p. 253), (245) (p. 414).

When answering item 25, users should look for confidence intervals applied to outcomes. The confidence level should be reported, e.g. 95%, 90% or 99%.

4.3.26. Is it clear how many participants were eligible, were enrolled, and were lost, excluded or had withdrawn?

This item relates to the internal and external validity of data. Knowing how many participants were enrolled and what the eligible population size was, assists readers in determining whether the sample was large enough and representative enough of the population under study. It is uncommon, however, to know the size of the eligible population. If many participants were lost or withdrew from the experiment, there may have been systematic factors at play, and these could render results biased. Lost participants (or data) are any that were allocated to an experimental group but not analysed, e.g. withdrawn or excluded participants and literally lost data. Withdrawn participants (or data) are those who removed themselves from the experiment after allocation. Excluded participants (or data) are removed by the investigators for any reason, e.g. outliers, non-compliance with the treatment.

Providing numbers of subjects who entered a study but were not part of statistical analysis allows readers to judge whether the final results are likely to be credible. This is particularly important for health informatics experimentation, which has adopted an intention to treat principle from medical experimentation (138) (p. 217), (146). Intention to treat analysis requires that all available data be analysed according to original group assignment (108). Poor or non-compliance with a treatment (whether a drug or the use of an information system) is not grounds for exclusion of a subject from analysis. It can lead to overestimates of the true benefit of an intervention in average use (138) (p. 217) and "bias associated with nonrandom loss of participants." (108)

When answering item 26, users should look for a description of the numbers of participants enrolled, lost, excluded or who had withdrawn and the size of the eligible population. A study that reports all applicable numbers should be marked highly.

4.3.27. What is the percentage of lost/withdrawn/excluded participants to the enrolled?

This item relates to internal and external validity. If a large number of enrolled participants or their data is not analysed then the remaining sample may not be representative of the population (108). There may also have been systematic reasons to have caused certain participants to have been lost to analysis, and this may bias the results (179).

When answering item 27, users should look for the number of enrolled participants and the number of those who were enrolled but who were not included in analysis. Reports often do not document percentage losses, and this must be calculated by hand. If adequate information cannot be found in the report, then the percentage cannot be calculated, and users should answer "unclear".

4.3.28. Are sample sizes calculated for all main outcomes?

Sample size calculations show the reader that the investigators have considered statistical power of their experiment as well as the estimated effect size and significance level (108, 166, 208). This is especially important for statistical nonsignificance of outcomes, which may be the consequence of insufficient power, i.e. type II error. The subtle interactions between informatics technologies/methods and humans may be similar to the situation in medical experimentation (108), (155) (p. 178), where small benefits of therapies require large numbers of participants, making assessment of power necessary.

When answering item 28, users should look for descriptions of sample size calculations for all main or primary outcomes. Ideally, all main outcomes have been assessed for sample size needed.

4.3.29. How appropriate is the use of scale type (level of measurement) e.g. nominal, ordinal, interval, ratio?

The level of measurement affects what statistical operations are appropriate, e.g. correct use of measures of central tendency and dispersion (153) (p. 82) and admissible transformations (269). There is, however, ongoing debate on the degree to which scale type affects statistical tests of inference (127, 128, 269) particularly when classifying scale type by parametric versus nonparametric tests (131) (p. 30), (153) (p. 95), (270) . Nevertheless, perhaps the most common mistake in informatics is treating ordinal data as continuous without justification, e.g. calculating the mean and standard deviation or applying inadmissible transformations like multiplication. Fenton provides the example "failure x is twice as critical as failure y" (16) when software failure criticality is probably ordinal rather than ratio. This is a particular problem in informatics where many metrics have not been shown to be beyond ordinal level (153) (p. 30). In health informatics, scale issues are less problematic than in other areas of informatics since many outcomes come from the medical domain and have well-understood properties, e.g. physiological measurements, population health rates, illness staging. However, mistakes still occur, such as the study by Cannon et al where nominal data (presence or absence of major depressive mood disorder and complete medical record documentation) were treated as interval (given a score of 0 or 1) for the purpose of analysis of variance (214).

When answering item 29, users should judge whether the data has been treated and interpreted in accordance with their scale type. If this was strictly not the case, then were such decisions reasonably justified?

4.3.30. How adequate is the description of the statistical tests used e.g. name, significance level, and corrections?

The statistical tests used should be documented since inappropriately used procedures can produce meaningless results. Basic requirements include the name of the test, e.g. t-test, Mann-Whitney test, ANOVA and level of significance (0.05, 0.1 etc). For rarely used statistical tests, investigators may need to describe them and how they apply to their experiment. Additionally any corrections to tests or data transformations should be documented.

When answering item 30, users should look for a statement about what statistical tests were employed. It should provide enough information to allow judgement of whether such tests were appropriate (items 31 and 34).

4.3.31. Are statistical test assumptions unacceptably violated?

If a statistical test's assumptions are violated, the results produced may be worthless, as interpretation may be impossible. Common assumptions include normal distribution of data and statistical independence of data. However, not all violations of assumptions are severe enough to render results uninterpretable. For instance, t-tests are robust against non-normality depending on the sample size and the presence of data outliers or strong skewness (245) (p. 463). In health informatics, statistical independence violations are common and cannot be tolerated by commonly used tests. Chuang et al's review of 24 studies found that 14 (58%) did not account for clustering, which can affect the independence of data, since participants within one cluster can be more related to each other than those between clusters (271). This can lead to unit of analysis error.

When answering item 31, users should judge whether statistical test violations have occurred and, if so, whether they have been severe enough to invalidate results.

4.3.32. Is unit of analysis error present (and not corrected for)?

The unit of analysis error occurs when statistical analysis does not consider independence of data. As Dallal states, "Measuring a single mouse 100 times is different from measuring 100 mice once each," because the former observations are more likely to be similar to each other than the latter observations are to each other (272). The units of analysis should be the smallest units that are independent of each other (272), which usually means one observation per participant (108). In other words, analysis should consider the level of treatment assignment such that the number of observations should match the number of units assigned treatment (273). The danger of unit of analysis error is type I error since p values and confidence intervals become artificially reduced (253).

Unit of analysis error is a particular problem for health informatics experiments but can potentially affect any naturally clustered data (98). Often patients are deemed the experimental unit, but their health care providers are allocated treatments. Unit of analysis will occur if, during statistical analysis, each patient is deemed a unit for analysis. This will occur because patients who attend a provider are probably more similar to others who attend the same provider than to those who attend another. The patients cluster around a provider and are therefore not independent of each other. As an interesting aside, it should be mentioned that this point is the same for many clinical drug trials, yet patients remain the unit of analysis (253). The reason for this illustrates the importance of unit of analysis in health informatics studies. In drug trials, strictly, patients who attend one hospital (most trials are conducted as single-centre studies) may be similar to each other than those who attend another hospital. Therefore, in a single-centre drug trial, the unit of analysis would be the hospital, yet analysis is nearly always performed on individual patient observations. This is accepted in drug trials because it is assumed that providers are all the same in their treatment of patients (253). That is, there is no provider-patient interaction (variance) for which to account. However, when the treatment affects provider care/behaviour, such as the assistance of a clinical information system, this can no longer be assumed.

Whiting-O'Keefe et al recommended two general approaches to address this problem. The first is to make providers the unit of analysis. The second is to create multivariate models that examine the patient-provider interactions (253), such as generalised linear models and estimating equations (274).

When answering item 32, users should judge whether data from samples are independent or clustered and whether statistical analyses has recognised this threat. If unit of analysis error was a threat, did the investigators use appropriate statistical techniques to address it?

4.3.33. Was a statistician consulted?

A statistical expert is likely to improve the quality of a controlled experiment. Such a person should be aware of pitfalls in the design and analysis of experiments and impart this knowledge to co-researchers. This item is related to internal and external validity. It is considered by the MICE index to be important to experimental quality because of the many ways in which an experiment can be poorly designed, conducted and analysed. Non-trivial experiments, i.e. most performed for publication in informatics journals, should have some expert input. This is especially important for complex or novel experimental designs.

In the last chapter, it was demonstrated as part of convergent construct validity testing that statistical assistance improves the quality of controlled experiments.

When answering item 33, users should look for an acknowledgement, or the like, of statistical assistance. This is sometimes presented in fine print. Alternatively, if it is clear that the investigators have statistical expertise, e.g. those from departments of statistics or epidemiology, or sometimes described in biographies, then this is acceptable.

4.3.34. How appropriate overall is the statistical analysis?

Statistical analysis is the second most important part of any controlled experiment (the first is experimental design since even faultless statistical analysis cannot save poor design.) Results from an experiment are the product of this process. Hence, if the process if flawed, results will be flawed and conclusions incorrect.

This is a highly abstracted item that calls for an overall judgement of statistical analysis. Answers to previous items can impact on this item. Furthermore, problems with statistical analysis not covered by previous items can be addressed here.

When answering item 34, users should judge whether any part of the process of statistical analysis could invalidate results.

4.3.35. To what extent are the investigators' conclusions justified?

Ultimately, the purpose of a controlled experiment is to produce conclusions based on rigorously examined data. Conclusions are perhaps the part of a report that is most remembered by readers, when the fine details of methodology and tables of results are long forgotten. Various poorly conducted aspects of the experiment can adversely affect this item. Any of the previous items may be considered again. Other aspects of the experiment not previously tapped but that affect the validity of conclusions will also determine how this item is answered.

Answering this item is also determined by the investigators' conclusions. Even if the experiment is performed perfectly, investigators may exaggerate their conclusions beyond what their data shows. Worse still is when conclusions are based more on rhetoric than data (275).

When answering item 35, users should judge whether any problems with the design, conduct and analysis of the experiment hamper the conclusions presented and whether conclusions are in keeping with the results.

4.3.36. How adequate is the discussion on how the findings relate to current evidence and/or theory?

To improve the relevancy of the results and conclusions of the experiment, investigators should relate these to the current state of knowledge. This assists readers in understanding the deficiency that the experiment tried to address and what the new findings add. If an experiment is novel and no body of evidence exists for the research question in mind, then ideally this should be stated. It is acceptable that an experiment can be exploratory in order to develop a hypothesis when no evidence exists, but this should be made known to readers.

Discussing the findings in terms of other evidence also builds the body of knowledge about a research hypothesis. No single experiment, however credible and applicable, is enough to make decisions about cause and effect relationships. Consistency with other studies is one of the criteria for deciding causation (245) (p. 178), (155) (p. 41). Comparison to other evidence is also important for systematic reviews and meta-analysis (108).

Similar to item 1, item 36 also has ethical implications in addition to quality concerns. When findings are compared to current knowledge, the Helsinki Declaration is supported (252).

When answering item 36, users should look for a discussion of how the findings confirm or refute the current state of knowledge. Alternatively, findings may be novel, but they should be related to some underlying theory.

4.3.37. How adequate is the discussion on external validity i.e. how the findings can be generalised?

External validity is the extent to which results can be generalised from the experiment to other populations, other settings and even other points in time (153) (p. 73). External validity is one of the common criticisms of controlled experimentation when compared to other empirical methods (276, 277). Results from controlled experiments may have greater internal validity than those from other forms of empirical research, but, because of the strict manipulation of variables, the results may only be applicable within the confines of that manipulation. A discussion on external validity is helpful to readers since they can determine whether the experimental findings apply to their own situation.

Depending on the research question and the design of the experiment, external validity may be restricted. A common issue in health informatics experiments is whether the benefit of an information system will be transferable to non-developer sites. The developer of a system often performs the evaluative controlled experiment. Therefore, there is a concern that developers provide users with extra support (278), and performance would be better than for sites without such champions. Similarly, tertiary academic hospitals are a common site due to university-based health informaticians and clinicians, but would results transfer to, for instance, a rural clinic (69)? In computer science, the frequent use of university student participants and laboratories, rather than professionals and real work places, may (or may not, depending on the research hypothesis) affect conclusions aimed at all computing practitioners.

When answering item 37, users should look for a discussion on external validity and judge whether investigators have correctly identified threats. If there is no discussion on possible threats to external validity, this item should be answered as "inadequate".

4.3.38. How adequately do the investigators discuss the limitations of the experiment?
Limitations are any problems or weaknesses with design, conduct and analysis of the experiment that could affect internal and external validity of results. This item requires that investigators acknowledge and report limitations of which they were aware. This item also inquires about limitations that went unnoticed or were unreported. All experimental reports should contain a description of real or potential threats. A description of experimental limitations helps readers to quickly identify caveats to the conclusions. Since no experiment is perfect, reporting the real or potential limitations of an experiment pays respect to the scientific method. Indeed, experimental trade-offs are common in research because resources (manpower, participants, funding, time etc) are not infinite. For example, as mentioned previously, a frequent potential limitation in computer science experimentation is the paucity of experimentation in real work places with computing professionals (91) due to the intrusiveness of such studies to industrial sites and the costliness of "hiring" participants (94).

When answering item 38, users may need to consider answers to previous items. Users should look for a treatise, preferably in the discussion section, about any problems that could limit the conclusions. If the investigators did not acknowledge a problem that could have adversely affected the experiment, this item should be marked down. If no discussion about limitations is present at all, this item should be answered as "inadequate". If investigators claim their experiment to be free of limitations (this would be bold), users should assess the claim. If in agreement, the item should be answered as "adequate". Otherwise, depending on the limitations identified, users should mark down the item accordingly.

4.4.   Discussion

This chapter presented the MICE-38 index questionnaire and explained the meanings of items and the rationales behind them. The research hypotheses stated that the instrument should be definable for informatics experiments. It is in examining the rationales that it becomes clear why certain experimental concepts need particular attention to in informatics (general and health). Some concepts will always be common to all experimental disciplines, such as the appropriate use of statistical methods, comparable experimental groups and justification of conclusions. However, because of the nature of informatics and the conduct of informatics experiments, some concepts need modification or different interpretation. Expectation effects and observer bias are particularly difficult problems because informatics is largely aimed at changing human information processing and metrics are largely judgment based. Creative methods are required for blinding in informatics; readers of reports need to consider their merits.

External validity in current computer science experimentation is a key quality problem and an area where computer science can learn from health informatics. Using real workers on real tasks in real environments is logistically challenging and expensive, but health informatics experiments are often conducted this way.

4.4.1.   Consideration of Categorical/Nominal Items

Level of measurement of items requires further discussion. This was raised in Chapter 2 with regards to the interval nature of experimental quality. Several items in the MICE index could be considered nominal, yet the responses are treated as continuous. Any item that contains an "unclear" response where clarity is not the construct being measured, e.g. items 15, 16 and 27, become nominal when such a response is added. This follows Sirkin's example (182), as shown in Box 1.

Strongly agree
Agree
Disagree
Strongly disagree
Unsure

Box 1. Sirkin's example of ordinal scales becoming nominal when the "logical sequence is broken." (182) (p. 42)

The aforementioned MICE-38 items measure reliability, validity and percentage data loss on an ordinal (and assumed interval) scale, but the addition of an "unclear" step makes them ordinal. Other items that do inquire about clarity, e.g. item 1's clarity of rationale, may include an "unclear" step and remain ordinal (or interval) because unclear is the lowest end of the spectrum. Items 19 and 20 may also be considered nominal since each response step could be considered to be a category, as well as any item that asks for a dichotomous yes/no response. As described in Chapter 2, nominal scale numerals are treated as labels; the numbers associated with response steps do not have permissible transformations other than 1-to-1 substitution. At first glance, summation of nominal values would appear to be inappropriate, like adding together football jersey numbers. In Chapter 2, the example of assigning 0 to males and 1 to females showed the labelling nature of nominal scales. However, if being female is to be "greater than" male, in some relationship, then it may make sense to assign value to gender. The key point is that, "Measurement is a process of assigning numbers to objects in such a way that *interesting qualitative empirical relations* among the objects are reflected in the numbers themselves as well as in important properties of the number system." (128) (italics added) It is the meaningful relation between objects that transforms the nominal into the ordinal. The nominal-appearing MICE items are ordinal because there is meaningful ranked order of quality. The presence of uncorrected unit of analysis error (item 32), for example, appears nominal in the sense that something is categorically present or not; it becomes ordinal because a yes response is deemed to indicate poorer experimental quality than a no response. Similarly, unknown reliability and validity (items 15 and 16) are assumed to have zero values and are, thus, lower than known poor reliability/validity.

The issue of nominal items being treated as ordinal/continuous is common to many of the medical scales discovered in this research. For instance the well-known Jadad scale is comprised of entirely dichotomous items, with affirmative responses given 1 point and negative responses given 0 points (141). MICE's item 27 can be compared to the similar items of the scales of Chalmers (142) and McMaster University (171). Chalmers item 2.3 for withdrawals provides the following responses in descending order of desirability: list given, no withdrawals, no list, unknown, >15% withdrawals for long-term studies and >10% for studies lasting less than 3 months. McMaster contains the following responses: outcome reported for at least 90% of patients starting the study, outcome reported for less than 90% but more than 80% of patients starting the study, outcome reported for less than 80% of patients starting the study. Both items have a point spread of 1 point between each response. At first it is apparently obvious that the Chalmers item is nominal (each response can be interpreted as an unordered category.) The McMaster item could also be considered purely categorical. However, it is in the qualitative empirical relation between each response (quality of experimental conduct with regards to managing data loss) that transforms these items into continuous measurement.

Another important issue is whether an interval or ratio nature of items can be justified. For data to be considered interval or ratio, the difference between values of an instrument reflect equal differences in what is being measured (185) (p. 10). For temperature, this means that the difference between 30 and 31 degrees Celsius is the same as the difference between 0 and 1 and that the difference of 1 degree always represents that same amount of heat. For quality instruments, is the difference between each item step (score) equal to the difference of amount of experimental quality? This is a potential weakness of all quality assessment scales because quality is difficult to understand in terms conceptual mapping to numbers. Like intelligence, quality and its rating scales must be assumed to be interval (185) (p. 10-11).

4.4.2. The Ratings Paradox

Lastly, the difference between scales that call for judgement versus ones that merely ask whether certain events had occurred should be discussed. The MICE index is defined for users with the ability to make appropriate judgement. Only a few items call for the simple noting of a quality issue, e.g. statistician assistance (item 33). In the early stages of MICE development, a decision was made to make the index more heavily weighted towards user judgment. As Friedman and Wyatt describe, this is the "art of measurement" in relation to this problem that they call the ratings paradox (138) (p. 179). With scales that only require simple observation, not judgement, reliability is increased, but the scales become "mechanical and possibly trivial" (have lower validity) (138) (p. 178). With greater judgement, rater reliability becomes important to establish, but the expertise of the judge is used and validity improves. The MICE index is believed to have managed the ratings paradox by having good reliability and validity, while being far from mechanical.

121

Chapter 5: An Application of the MICE Index

5.1. Introduction

Chapters 3 and 4 dealt with the creation and content of the MICE index and described how the research hypotheses were fulfilled. This chapter supports the research hypotheses by applying the index to review the quality of health informatics trials of clinical decision support tools and clinical decision support systems (CDSS). It provides an example of how the MICE index can be used to conduct quantitative systematic reviews of controlled experiments in informatics. This is especially important for general informatics where reviews of experiments and their quality have yet to be published in the fashion of the McMaster University series (112). However, even in health informatics, there is still a need to continually assess the quality of trials, to see trends (154) and understand where they could be improved. As with all improvement, the first step is quantification.

The MICE index could be used to establish and monitor experimental quality in informatics and thus is a valuable contribution to the field, but a caveat is that the same version should be applied consistently. This is important because scores from different versions, such as MICE-38 and MICE-80 (and future incarnations of the index) may not be directly comparable. The MICE index may remain reliable and valid when items are removed or modified, but final scores can be affected depending on each study's responses to the items that are changed. This can be demonstrated by the difference between mean scores of studies assessed in Chapter 3 as part of reliability tests. Mean scores fell after reducing the 80-item index to 38 items by 0.054 points (95% CI 0.040 - 0.067, df = 57, p = 0.000) from 0.573 to 0.519 (paired samples t-test).

The MICE index can be further applied to weight results from studies according to experimental quality for the purpose of meta-analysis and should be the subject of further research.

This review is not intended to be comprehensive but to illustrate how the index could be used. Therefore, only the reports published for clinical decision support tools for the year 2007 are examined. However, a larger assessment of experimental quality in health informatics could be performed, as could an assessment of general computer science experiments. Because of the large number of reports published over many years, endeavours such as these would require the availability of several reviewers using the MICE index. A small review such as this, however, does add to the field of health informatics by being current. It is, to the author's knowledge, the most recent evaluation of trials of clinical decision support tools using a quality measurement scale.

Controlled experimentation in health informatics is, of course, not limited to summative assessment of decision support tools. Indeed, in informatics in general, one can utilise human experimentation in formative, summative and scientific roles and for various informatics objects and methods. In Chapter 1, the influence of medicine on experimental evaluation in health informatics was noted. It is thus common to see summative trials of informatics products in the fashion of trials of medical therapies. Hence, this small review focuses on summative experiments. Additionally, decision support tools are not the only objects to evaluate in health informatics, whether by controlled trial or other evaluation method. This small review chooses decision support tools because experimental evaluation of them is the typical health informatics experiment, as shown by the McMaster University reviews (112).

However, experimentation in health informatics can also be used to establish evidence for scientific theory. Not only is it important for tools to be shown to be effective when those effects may be difficult to appreciate, but the correct circumstances or properties of tools that lead to successful use can be determined by experiment. Kawamoto et al (279), for instance, examined CDSS trials to determine such technical and informational features. Such efforts produce a body of scientific knowledge that informs the future development and appropriate usage of informatics objects.

5.2.   Method

The health informatics literature was searched to retrieve reports of controlled experiments (trials) of clinical decision support tools. Table 34 lists the journal and conference sources and search strategies. Journal and conference proceeding sources were obtained from 2 main resources: PubMed (The US National Library of Medicine, Bethesda, USA) and health informatics journals listed in Journal Citation Reports 2006 edition (The Thompson Corporation, Stamford, USA). In addition to using the PubMed online search function, the search functions of online journals where available were used. Only reports published in year 2007 and in English were eligible. A trial was eligible if there was an intervention and control group, but there was no requirement for controls to be parallel, in keeping with the design of the MICE index. Trials were required to be completed, i.e. with results and a discussion. Therefore, plans for trials or those underway without reportable results were excluded. Pilot trials were included if they had produced results. A clinical decision support tool was defined as an electronic computer-based aid that processed patient-specific data to produce recommendations or advice to its user for the purpose of improving decision making. This definition follows ones commonly found in the health informatics literature, e.g. (79, 183). Therefore, this excluded simple reproduction of paper-based content in electronic form (e.g. websites, digital media etc). Users were not restricted only to health care providers to allow for consumer (patient) informatics tools. Monitoring and telecare devices were excluded, as were medical imaging technologies if they did not provide advice or recommendations to health care providers. Where it was unclear from the abstract whether a trial was eligible, it was retrieved as a full-text document and read.

Source	Search strategy	Search engine
American Medical Informatics Association Annual Symposia	(no 2007 proceedings)	PubMed search
PubMed	decision support system clinical + clinical trial (MeSH terms)	PubMed search
PubMed	"decision support" + "trial"	PubMed search
JCR health informatics sources		
Artificial Intelligence in Medicine	"trial"	Journal search
Computer Methods and Programs in Biomedicine	"trial"	Journal search
Computers Informatics Nursing	"trial"	Journal search
IEEE Engineering in Medicine and Biology	"trial"	Journal search
IEEE Transactions on Information Technology in Biomedicine	"trial"	Journal search
International Journal of Medical Informatics	"trial"	Journal search
International Journal of Technology Assessment in Healthcare	"trial"	Journal search
Journal of Biomedical Informatics	"trial"	Journal search
Journal of Medical Internet Research	"trial"	Journal search
Journal of Medical Systems	"trial"	Journal search
Journal of the American Medical Informatics Association	"trial"	Journal search
Medical Decision Making	"trial"	Journal search
Methods of Information in Medicine	"trial"	PubMed search

Table 34. Journal and conference proceedings sources used for the review of controlled trials of clinical decision support tools.

MeSH: Medical Subject Heading; JCR: Journal Citation Reports.

Trials were evaluated with MICE-38 by the author. Intra and inter-rater reliability were not assessed. Statistical analysis was performed using SPSS 15 (SPSS Inc., Chicago, USA), Microsoft Excel 2000 (Microsoft, Seattle, USA) and Researcher's Toolkit (DSS Research, Fort Worth, USA) (280). Statistical significance was defined at an alpha of 0.05.

Item means were analysed to see where methodological problems in the conduct of the trials arose. For each of the 38 items, the values from the 21 eligible studies were averaged and then standardised by dividing by the maximum possible value and multiplying by 100. Items that had a standardised response of less than 50% were a priori defined as indicating areas of trial conduct that need quality improvement.

To further assess the usefulness of validity tests described in Chapter 3, the same techniques were applied to this sample of studies. The exception was known-groups testing using the McMaster University scale to dichotomise studies into high and low quality, since the sample of studies in this

2007 review had not been assessed by the McMaster panel of experts using their scale. The other exception was the divergent construct validity test of publication year, since all papers were from 2007. Hence, the convergent hypothetical construct that statistician (or equivalent) assistance should lead to higher MICE scores was tested against this 2007 sample. Also, the divergent hypothetical constructs that the number of authors, cited references and page length should not be related to MICE scores were tested against this 2007 sample. Finally, for criterion validity, MICE scores for this 2007 sample were assessed against the Journal Impact Factor (2006 edition) of their journals.

5.3.   Results

29 reports of controlled trials of clinical decision support tools were found using the search strategy. 8 reports were ineligible as shown in Table 35.

First author	Decision support tool	Reason for ineligibility
Bosworth (281, 282)	Blood pressure home telecare system with generated recommendations	Plan for trial
Holbrook (283)	Computer programme explaining risks and benefits of anticoagulation therapies	No patient-specific data processing
Krist (284)	Website page explaining prostate specific antigen screening	No patient-specific data processing
Saver (285)	Website explaining risks and benefits of hormone replacement therapy	Unclear whether patient specific data used
Shulman (286)	Computerised protocol advising on insulin therapy for intensive care patients	Uncontrolled observational study
van Steenkiste (287)	Booklet informing patients on cardiovascular risk	Non-computerised aid
Zwarenstein (288)	Electronic prescribing software which checks for drug dosing and interaction errors	Plan for trial

Table 35. References returned by the search process but considered ineligible.

21 trials of clinical decision support tools were eligible for evaluation by MICE-38 and are summarised in Table 36.

Systems ranged from standalone applications on personal digital assistants (PDA) (289) to hospital-wide information systems (e.g. order entry systems) (290) and addressed a range of clinical problems for health care providers (13/21) and patients (8/21).

The mean MICE-38 score was 0.656 (95% CI 0.583 - 0.729) (N = 21), with a median of 0.704 and standard deviation of 0.160. Raw item values are presented in Appendix D. The distribution of scores was approximately bell-shaped and skewed to the left, as shown by Figure 23. This is

First author	Decision support tool	User	MICE-38 score
Albisser (291)	Telemedical centralised database predicting diabetic patient hypoglycaemia	Physician	0.614
Augstein (292)	Metabolism/therapy simulator advising on patient diabetic management	Physician	0.648
Col (293)	Computerised risk assessment for patients facing hormone replacement therapy decisions	Patient	0.803
Davis (294)	Electronic prescription writer providing prescribing advice for common childhood illnesses	Physician	0.782
Davison (295)	Computer programme providing individualised information for men with prostate cancer	Patient	0.754
Emery (296)	Computer programme assessing risk of familial cancers	Physician	0.776
Glassman (297)	Computerised provider order entry system with a drug review component to reduce adverse drug events	Physician	0.636
Kaner (298) §	Computer programme providing individualised risks and benefits of anticoagulation therapies	Patient	0.585
Leibovici (299)	Hospital computer programme advising on antibiotic treatments for common infections	Physician	0.369
Martens (300)	Primary care information system advising on appropriate drug prescribing for asthma, chronic obstructive airways disease and antibiotics	Physician	0.737
Momtahan (289)	PDA programme for triage and management of chest pain	Nurse	0.229
Montgomery (301)	Computer programme advising on mode of delivery for pregnant women with previous caesarian section	Patient	0.740
Ozanne (302)	Computer programme assessing risk of breast cancer	Patient	0.631
Peterson (303)	Computerised provider order entry system for reducing adverse drug events among the elderly	Physician	0.363
Protheroe (304)	Computer programme advising on treatment of menorrhagia	Patient	0.856
Raebel (305)	Computerised provider order entry system for reducing pregnancy-drug interactions	Physician	0.631
Reeve (306)	Pharmacy dispensing software advising on aspirin therapy for eligible diabetic patients	Pharmacist	0.704
Rothschild (290)	Computerised provider order entry system advising on appropriate blood product transfusion	Physician	0.631
Schapira (307)	Computerised risk assessment for patients facing hormone replacement therapy decisions	Patient	0.790
Taylor (308)	Emergency department information system advising on asthma management	Physician	0.744
Thompson (309) §	Computer programme providing individualised risks and benefits of anticoagulation therapies	Patient	0.756

Table 36. Summary of references returned by the search strategy, the user of the decision support tool and MICE-38 scores.

§: These systems were the same but evaluated in different trials with different objectives and outcomes.

supported by a significant Sharpiro Wilks test (p = 0.003) and a skewness to standard error ratio of <-2 (Table 37). The 3 scores (Leibovici, Momtahan, Peterson) in the left tail were possible outliers (<1st quartile minus 1.5 times the interquartile range). These studies were examined again for data input error (MICE questionnaire completion errors), and this was not the reason for outlier behaviour. Table 37 shows summary data including and excluding outliers. Since the reason for outlier behaviour is unknown, outliers were included in analysis. The effect of the outliers on central tendency and dispersion of the sample was not great.

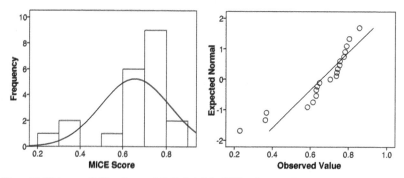

Figure 23. Histogram (left) and normal Q-Q plot of the 2007 review sample.

	Outliers included	Outliers excluded
N	21	18
Mean	.656	.712
95% CI for mean	.583 - .729	.673 - .751
Median	.704	.739
Standard deviation	.160	.079
Skewness (SE)	-1.431 (.501)*	-.041 (.536)
Kurtosis (SE)	1.700 (0.972)	-1.195 (1.038)
Shapiro Wilks statistic	.843	.930
Shapiro Wilks p	.003*	.191

Table 37. Summary data for 2007 review sample including and excluding outliers.
*: non-normality; SE: standard error.

Nevertheless, statistical tests on the whole sample are conservatively based on non-normal distributions. When the outliers are removed, the distribution is approximately normal as shown in Figure 24 and supported by other measures of normality (Shapiro Wilks test, skewness and kurtosis analysis) (Table 37).

Item response means are presented in Table 38 with the median response and standardised value. Standardised means are also plotted in Figure 25. Median responses were similar to mean responses. Questionnaire items 2, 13, 17, 20, 21, 22, 33 and 35 had standardised responses less than 50%.

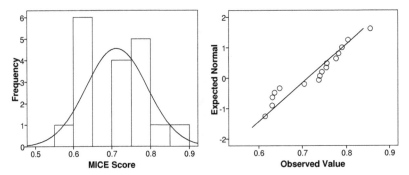

Figure 24. Histogram (left) and normal Q-Q plot of the 2007 review sample excluding outliers.

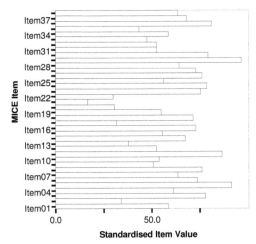

Figure 25. Bar chart of standardised means for each item for the 2007 review.

Studies correlated poorly with their journal's JIF. 16/21 studies had corresponding JIF's in the Journal Citation Reports 2006 edition. The Spearman rho correlation coefficient was −0.167 (Table 39), and the scatterplot showed no obvious relationship (Figure 26).

When testing the convergent construct validity hypothesis of statistical assistance, scores were recomputed without item 33 (statistical assistance item) as inclusion of the item increases the difference between the two groups (see Chapter 3.) Groups with and without assistance were found

Item	Mean response	Median response	Standardised mean
1	3.52	4	58.73
2*	2.05	1	34.13*
3	4.67	5	77.78
4	3.67	4	61.11
5	5.48	5	91.27
6	4.43	4	73.81
7	3.81	4	63.49
8	4.57	6	76.19
9	3.05	3	50.79
10	3.24	4	53.97
11	5.19	5	86.51
12	0.52	1	52.38
13*	0.38	0	38.10*
14	4.05	4	67.46
15	3.33	4	55.56
16	4.38	5	73.02
17*	0.95	0	31.75*
18	4.29	5	71.43
19	1.64	2	54.76
20*	0.92	0	30.56*
21*	0.33	0	16.67*
22*	0.60	0	30.00*
23	4.52	6	75.40
24	4.71	5	78.57
25	3.38	5	56.35
26	4.57	5	76.19
27	2.19	3	73.02
28	1.29	2	64.29
29	5.76	6	96.03
30	4.76	6	79.37
31	0.52	1	52.38
32	0.52	1	52.38
33*	0.48	0	47.62*
34	3.52	3	58.73
35*	2.62	3	43.65*
36	4.86	6	80.95
37	4.10	5	68.25
38	3.81	4	63.49

Table 38. Mean, median and standardised mean for each item response of the 2007 review. (N=21). *: Items with a standardised response <50%.

	N	Rho	p
JIF	16	-.167	.536
Authors	21	.044	.850
References	21	.163	.481
Pages	21	.254	.267

Table 39. Spearman rho correlations between 2007 review MICE-38 scores and Journal Impact Factors, number of study authors, cited references and page count.

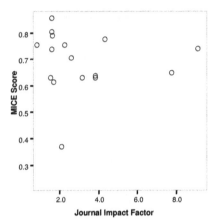

Figure 26. Scatterplot of 2007 review MICE-38 scores vs. study Journal Impact Factor.

to have approximately normal distributions of scores as shown in Table 40, Figure 27 and Figure 28.

	Statistician-assisted group	Statistician-unassisted group
Skewness (SE)	-.399 (.687)	-.843 (.661)
Kurtosis (SE)	-1.682 (1.334)	-.442 (1.279)
Shapiro-Wilks statistic	.875	.896
Shapiro-Wilks df	10	11
Shapiro-Wilks p	.116	.163

Table 40. Measures of normality for the statistician-assisted and unassisted groups in the 2007 review sample.

SE: standard error.

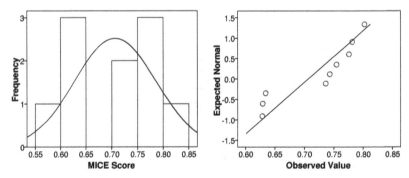

Figure 27. Histogram (left) and normal Q-Q plot of the statistician-assisted group from 2007 review sample.

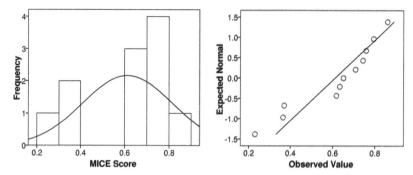

Figure 28. Histogram (left) and normal Q-Q plot of the statistician-unassisted group from 2007 review sample.

A 2-tailed independent samples t-test was used to assess the MICE-38 scores. The statistical assistance group had a higher mean MICE-38 score than the unassisted group (difference 0.094). However, the result did not reach significance due to insufficient sample size as indicated by the wide confidence interval (95% CI −0.048 - 0.237). Post-hoc power analysis, as recommended by Chalmers et al (142), showed the power to be low at 33% (280). Results are summarised in Table 41 and Table 42.

Statistician	N	Mean MICE score	Standard deviation
Yes	10	.707	.079
No	11	.612	.202

Table 41. Descriptive statistics for the effect of statistical assistance on 2007 review sample MICE-38 scores.

	Levene's test		t-test (2-tailed)			
	F	p	t	df	p	Mean difference (95% CI)
Equal variances assumed	5.455	.031	1.376	19	.185	.094 (−.049 - .238)
Equal variances not assumed			1.428	13.232	.177	.094 (−.048 - .237)

Table 42. 2-tailed independent samples t-test results comparing the MICE-38 scores from 2007 review studies that had and did not have statistical assistance.

Divergent construct validity tests showed poor Spearman rho correlations between study MICE-38 scores and author, reference and page counts (Table 39). No strong scatterplot relationships can be seen in Figure 29.

5.4.   Discussion

This review of clinical decision support tools published in 2007 demonstrates one application of the

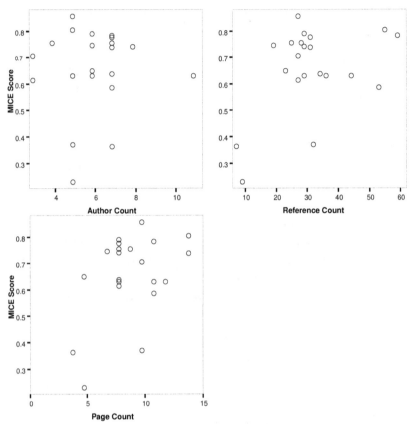

Figure 29. Scatterplots of 2007 review MICE-38 scores vs. studies' number of authors, references and pages.

MICE index: to assess and monitor the methodological quality of controlled experiments for summative evaluation of computerised tools. This is a common reason for performing controlled experiments in health informatics. In a recent Cochrane review regarding the assessment of clinical decision support systems, it was written, "It is clear that the bottom line is improvement to either patient outcomes, or physician performance. Indeed, improvement in these outcomes is precisely the raison d'etre (sic) for CDSS." (79) The McMaster University series is a good example of this view of experimental evaluation in health informatics (112, 171, 183). This series monitored such outcomes, as well as methodological quality of the summative trials. Such work is important to informatics in general. While summative evaluation is common in health informatics, in principle, it can be applied to other fields of informatics and information tools. An example is one of the summative experiments encountered in this research: a "collaboratory" electronic tool for improving teamwork among scientific researchers (206). The importance of high quality computer science experimentation has been noted, as shown by the development of published guidelines (Table 3); reviews of quality are present in the literature, e.g. (91). The MICE index can further quantitative assessments in computer science experiments and allow researchers to publish reviews in the manner of McMaster University.

5.4.1. Areas of High Quality in Clinical Decision Support Tool Experiments

The quality of 21 papers reporting controlled experiments of clinical decision support systems in 2007 was fair to good. Despite the presence of potential outliers skewing the sample to the left, the mean MICE-38 score was 0.656 (95% CI 0.583 - 0.729, median 0.704). A score of 50% is a reasonable threshold for defining high and low quality studies, since the mean of the 58 studies used to test MICE-38 in Chapter 3 was 0.519 (standard error = 0.047, median 0.519). Some aspects of experimental conduct were performed very well. Most treatments were suitable to the experimental questions being considered by investigators (item 5, standardised mean 91.27). Participants were usually taken from the "real world" and usually highly representative (item 11, standardised mean 86.51). This is a particular experimental issue handled well in health informatics that computer science experiments involving human participants can learn from, since external validity with student participants can be problematic (94). It is often argued that performing controlled experiments with computing professionals has logistical and motivational difficulties (94, 159). However, similar difficulties can apply to health care provider and patient samples. Yet, in health informatics, computerised tools are usually designed to assist working professionals, and controlled experiments involving students (unless they were indistinguishable from professionals in important ways) would be criticised for poor external validity. Item 29, inquiring about appropriate use of measurement scale, was highly scored (standardised mean 96.03). Scale types are perhaps more established in health informatics than other areas of informatics. For example, some of the outcomes measured in this review were blood glucose, adverse drug event counts and patient decisional conflict, and these are quite well understood in terms of level of measurement. Finally, report discussions brought the findings back to current evidence and theory quite well (item 36, standardised mean 80.95). This is important because health informatics is a young field that needs to build a strong evidence base (135). Even the large review of Garg et al (112) could not provide definitive advice on the effects of clinical decision support systems on patient outcomes (only about half the studies assessed patient outcomes and many of them with low statistical power.) When there are few studies on a particular topic in informatics, it is important to relate findings in order to build a body of evidence.

5.4.2.   Areas of Poor Quality in Clinical Decision Support Tool Experiments

Overall papers were of fair to good quality, but some methodological practices were done poorly (a priori defined as <50% standardised item mean). Item 2 called for clearly stated null and/or alternative hypotheses (standardised mean 34.13). Many studies gave broad objectives and not precise hypotheses. One possible reason is that controlled experiments in biomedicine are so established that the provision of formal hypotheses is considered too elementary. Nevertheless, hypothesis statements are clear, concise and easy to locate in a report. Furthermore, there is an expectation in computer science experimentation guidelines (113, 114, 122, 159, 166, 167) that they be used. Allocation concealment was not performed often enough (standardised mean 38.1). As described in Chapter 4, allocation concealment is important to avoid subversion of subject allocation, which can lead to systematic bias. Infrequent use of allocation concealment was also found in Garg et al's review (28% of 88 trials) (112) and remains an area for improvement in health informatics experiments. This is also likely to be a problem area for general informatics experiments (none of the experimental computing guidelines used to create MICE discussed allocation concealment as a concept.) Responses to item 17 showed that most study outcomes were subjective (standardised mean 31.75). This is the result of several reports of consumer informatics applications, which measured the effect of the tools on patient decisional conflict and decisional satisfaction (295, 298, 301, 302, 304, 307, 309). Subjective measures can suffer from reliability and validity problems, but, in this group of studies, a tested questionnaire for measuring decisional conflict was applied (310). Contamination effects (item 20, standardised mean 30.56) were a problem among the 2007 sample. None of the studies were of crossover design hence there were no crossover effects. Normally contamination occurs when decision support is given at the patient level where treating providers can be exposed to both treatment and control participants. However, one study in the 2007 sample provides another view of contamination. Rothschild et al (290) allocated interventions at the physician level but not to all physicians. Only junior doctors (32% of total hospital physicians) were allocated to the decision support group (assisted blood product transfusion) or control group. The remaining 68% were more senior doctors, who were assigned control state. However, transfusion decisions were made as medical teams, consisting of junior and senior doctors, and the senior colleagues commonly overrode decisions. To avoid such contamination of treatment and control effects, allocation should occur at team level. Blinding of participants and outcome assessors was poor (items 21, 22, standardised means 16.67, 30). Blinding of participants to informatics technologies is tremendously difficult, and in this series several studies examined the educational effects of a decision support tool on personal decisional conflict. Blinding in these cases is not possible because the potential benefit of the tool is clearly apparent, as is its use. Expectation effects may well have clouded some of the treatment effect. In such cases, care must be taken by investigators not to overemphasise the potential benefits of decision support tools to participants if blinding is not achievable. Unfortunately, tools were not sophisticated enough to provide selective exposure to an informational intervention to counter expectations, as described in (263). Blinding of outcome assessors is usually much easier but was mostly unreported or not done. As with participant blinding, this is important to avoid systematic bias. Statistical expert involvement (or equivalent) was moderate (item 33, standardised mean 47.62). This can be a problem as controlled experiments in health informatics can be complex with several methodological pitfalls. The methodological issues described above and some that missed the threshold, e.g. item 10 (appropriate experimental unit level, standardised mean 53.97) and item 12 (completely randomised allocation, standardised mean 52.38), meant that experimental findings were to be interpreted with caution (item 35, standardised mean 43.65). This is not incongruent with the overall MICE-38 mean of 0.656 because the MICE score incorporates reporting as well as methodological concerns. Item 35 also depends on how the investigators have interpreted their findings and whether they have extrapolated beyond what their data shows.

Finally, two further issues should be visited as areas of improvement. As mentioned above, randomisation procedures were described only modestly well. The MICE index penalises reports that do not include a description of randomisation method, such as computer or table-generated, since some methods, which are believed to be random, may actually suffer from important systematic influence. Garg et al's review (112) found that 52% described a random method, which is the same finding of this review (item 12). Because of the known effect of nonrandomised allocation on experimental results (see Chapter 4), it should be mandatory that randomisation methods be clearly documented (108). The second issue is statistical independence of data. In Chuang et al's sample of CDSS experiments (271), 58% of studies accounted for clustered data in the analysis. In Garg et al's sample 40% used a cluster as the unit of analysis or adjusted for clustering in analysis. In this 2007 sample of CDSS experiments, unit of analysis error was not appreciably present or was corrected for in 52% (item 32). It would appear that Chuang et al's concern 7 years ago that many health informaticians are not aware of clustering issues is still applicable.

5.4.3. MICE Validation Tests and Review Data
The methods used to test the MICE index's validity in Chapter 3 are novel. Previous scales in health informatics had not tested the validity of their instruments. No adequate external criteria for

informatics experimental quality exist. There has not been sufficient research in understanding the nature of experimental quality in informatics. Chapter 3 discussed how the MICE index's validity tests contributed to psychometric evaluation of experimental quality scales. However, ideas should be tested on further examples to build a body of evidence. To this end, validity tests from Chapter 3 were applied again to this set of 2007 health informatics experiments, where they could be applied. The use of Journal Impact Factor as a form of criterion validity was again not supported by this sample. In Chapter 3, using the MICE-38 questionnaire version, Spearman rho correlation between scores and JIF was 0.297. In this 2007 sample, Spearman rho was −0.167. Scatterplots (Figure 21 and Figure 26) showed poor relationships. Hence, these samples provide some evidence against Journal Impact Factor as a proxy for experimental quality. The other form of criterion validity testing used in Chapter 3, i.e. known-groups testing, was not performed since the 2007 sample was not delineated by an external standard into high and low quality studies (in Chapter 3, the McMaster University review panel and scale achieved this through the paper by Garg et al (112).) Known-groups testing is, however, established as a method of validity testing (125) (p. 54). Further work to test the applicability of known-groups tests would require assembling an expert panel to categorise studies prior to application of the MICE-38 questionnaire. Because of the limitation of access to such a panel, this work was not performed; it remains to be the subject of future validity tests.

Of the construct validity tests used in Chapter 3, all but the correlation between publication year and MICE-38 score were repeated with the 2007 sample. The convergent hypothesis that MICE scores should improve with the assistance of a statistical expert was not supported due to statistical nonsignificance (p = 0.177). The 95% CI for the mean difference was wide (−0.048 to 0.237) but suggests that the convergent relationship was present and that the 2007 sample size was inadequate. A power of only 33% was achieved. A problem with this review was that it was not adequately designed to examine the convergent hypothesis. A sample size calculation was not performed since the objective of the review was to demonstrate an application of the MICE index to 2007 papers. A larger sample would have probably demonstrated the effect of statistical expert assistance. The divergent hypothesis tests were supported by the 2007 sample. The Spearman correlations between number of study authors, cited references and pages were weak (0.044 to 0.254, 2007 sample vs. −0.038 to 0.149, validity tests sample) without obvious scatterplot patterns.

Although some of the criterion and construct validity tests repeated in this review support the tests applied in Chapter 3, a body of evidence accumulates from constant research. Hence, future tests with the MICE index using different samples and different researchers should occur.

The finding that the overall 2007 sample had a left-skewed distribution of MICE-38 scores does not agree with the finding of a roughly normal distribution of study scores in Chapter 3 (Figure 14). This was the result of 3 low outliers, which could not be explained. Since not enough is known about the distribution of experimental quality in informatics, researchers should routinely plot their data and perform normality tests. Similarly, outliers should be treated conservatively unless there is an obvious reason for exclusion. The use of robust statistical tests and large sample sizes does not permit ignorance about distributions of quality when they are largely unknown.

5.4.4. Further Definitional Issues for CDSS

This review also raises an issue in health informatics that is worthy of mention, though it deserves a deeper discussion elsewhere. Some articles were returned under the National Library of Medicine's Medical Subject Heading (MeSH) definition of clinical decision support system that did not exactly meet that definition. The definition of a CDSS under the MeSH controlled vocabulary is, "Computer-based information systems used to integrate clinical and patient information and provide support for decision-making in patient care." (311) This implies computational processing of patient-specific data and therefore excludes, for instance, web-based publication of paper-based material. Yet, a few of the articles were ineligible in this review because of lack of patient data processing. For example, the report by Holbrook et al (283) described the evaluation of 3 decision aids to assist patients with atrial fibrillation about anti-coagulation therapy decisions: a decision board, a booklet with audiotape and an interactive computer programme. However, the computer programme did not use the individual patient's medical data. Rather, "Identical information was included in each type of decision aid." Similarly the web-based decision aid by Krist et al (284) is simply an online document (http://www.acorn.fap.vcu.edu/psa) without patient data computation.

The definition of decision support systems can become blurred in clinical medicine, as opposed to other domains where decision supporting information systems are used. Liu et al (312) for instance define "decision tools" as objects that assist in decision making, linked together by a common health technology assessment perspective, rather than a technical perspective. Therefore, they argue, patient information leaflets and predictive scores, such as the Glasgow Coma Scale, should be considered alongside information systems. The rationale for this blurring is justified in medicine and, by association, in health informatics for 2 reasons: evaluation of various decision aids that support decision making is, as Liu et al rightly point out, conceptually the same; if cheaper and more accessible decision aids produce the same clinical outcomes then ethical use of resources compels the use of simpler alternatives. In this sense, the reports of Holbrook and Krist were appropriately published under the keyword of decision support system, even though the MeSH definition does not fit.

137

The consistency with which people in health informatics interpret "decision support system" needs further examination. Since many controlled experiments in health informatics involve decision support systems, this is a related issue to this research but is beyond its scope.

5.4.5. Issues in Consumer Informatics Experiments

Another issue raised by this review is the rise of consumer health informatics. In Garg et al's review (112), none of the systems were aimed at the consumer (patient). Systems in their paper were categorised into systems for diagnosis, prevention, disease management and drug dosing and prescribing (health care provider activities). With growing consumer use of the Internet and informatics technologies for health care information (313) and the poor level of evidence concerning the advantages and disadvantages (314), high quality empirical (experimental) evaluation will be needed. The large proportion of experiments concerning consumer informatics applications in this review may be revealing a trend towards creating an experimental evidence base. However, methodological issues must still be remembered. For example, the interpretation of unit of analysis error in consumer health decision support experiments can be difficult. Generally, unit of analysis error occurs when health care providers are allocated the informatics intervention, which modifies their clinical performance, but their patients are considered the unit for analysis. Because patient outcomes are probably clustered around provider performance, statistical analysis should occur at the provider level. With consumer informatics interventions, the degree of clustering around a provider can be difficult to tell. These technologies aim to improve a patient's knowledge of health in order to facilitate decision making regarding her own circumstances. Consumer informatics technologies can therefore be aimed solely at the patient (arming the patient with knowledge to then take to her provider in a future consultation) or at the provider to use with the patient. In the former, one can probably ignore any unit of analysis problems because the provider-patient interaction can be ignored. This is akin to ignoring the provider-patient interaction when a physician gives a medication during a drug trial (in the words of Whiting O'Keefe et al, providers could be assumed "interchangeable." (253)). In the latter, the performance of the provider probably cannot be ignored (providers no longer interchangeable with respect to a certain outcome). Hence, the difficulty arises when it is not clearly reported or understood how much provider interaction with the patient and technology occurs.

Chapter 6: Conclusion

6.1. Summary

The controlled experiment is a useful method to acquire knowledge in computer science and health informatics. In the first chapter, questions about how humans benefit from informational resources, such as information systems, communications technologies and even simple pieces of paper, can be answered by performing experiments. In what situations can complex information technologies be replaced by simpler technologies? What are the factors that predict the best use of information resources? Experiments can also be applied to understand how to improve the development of information technologies. The benefits of computer-based tools are dependent upon them working as intended. In the subdiscpline of software engineering, large software failures have prompted a plethora of ideas on how to improve software quality. Accompanying the ideas has been a voice of reason asking proponents to question how they know the ideas work; this voice of reason is empiricism and experimentation. So, in as much as experimentation can help to answer what the benefits of informatics objects are, it can also help us to be more scientific in how we develop them and how we use them.

Experimentation and positivism are some of the tools at the disposal of informatics researchers. They sit amongst other methods and philosophies, which have their roles in computing and informatics research. Even "hard-nosed" computer scientists, interested in computability and hardware engineering and who may not see the importance of experiments, must realise that humans are always involved in computing. The controlled experiment is a rigorous way of understanding the relationships between humans and computing. This idea is commonplace in health informatics, where clinical evaluation is important, and is growing in computer science.

Whatever research methods are used, they must be done to satisfactory standards. This has been recognised in medicine with official guidelines on how to conduct and publish controlled trials and endorsement of guidelines by major medical journals. One sees similar efforts in health informatics and computer science to improve the quality of controlled experiments and other types of empirical study.

The high-level goal of this research is to improve experimental quality. The first step is to measure it; one cannot know without measuring. The research hypotheses were that:

- A reliable and valid questionnaire instrument for measuring experimental quality could be developed for human-based experiments in informatics.

139

- The instrument could be applied to computer science experiments.

- The instrument could be applied to health informatics experiments.

Such work had not been done in computer science, and instruments in health informatics were unsatisfactory due to questionable reliability and lack of formal validity testing (see p. 56-59.) The example of medical trial quality instruments was a source of inspiration.

However, it was predicted and discovered that medical trial quality is not the same as informatics experimental quality, even for health informatics. The construct of experimental quality has also not been researched in the informatics literature. What is experimental quality? What are its properties? Psychometrics provides useful theory for understanding and measuring things that are not easily observable.

Psychometric scale development methods were used to create an initial 80-item questionnaire: the MICE-80 index. MICE-80 was based on 40 literature sources from computer science, health informatics and medicine (see p. 57.); they were used to generate over 200 experimental concepts or practice tips important to quality (see Appendix A.) To test score consistency, the MICE-80 questionnaire was applied to 58 computer science and health informatics experimental studies (see p. 65-66.) This was performed 3 times under the method of test-retest; the reliability (intraclass correlation) coefficient was 0.935 (95% CI 0.884 - 0.962) (p. 64-68). The face and content validity of the MICE-80 index was assumed, but formal methods, some of which novel, for testing criterion and construct validity were applied. Because no gold standards against which the MICE index could be tested existed, a known-groups approach using studies previously judged in a systematic review was used (p. 74). The MICE-80 index was shown to be able to discriminate between poor and good studies, as judged by the review; good studies scored about 12% higher than poor ones (95% CI 4 - 19, $p = 0.004$) (p. 75). Journal Impact Factor is currently being assessed as an indicator of clinical trial quality in medical research. This research questioned whether JIF were related to MICE index scores; the MICE-80 scores correlated poorly (Pearson $r = 0.329$) (p. 75-75). Construct validity tests were completely new, since no previous work had been done in computer science or health informatics. The convergent hypothesis that statistician assistance in the experiment should increase MICE-80 scores was supported; scores were higher by 10% (95% CI 5 - 15, $p = 0.000$) (p. 76-77). The divergent hypotheses that quality is unrelated to the number of authors, cited references and pages and year of publication were also supported, as shown by absolute Pearson correlations of <0.2 (p. 78).

The MICE-80 version was reduced to 38 items using 3 criteria: item non-response >5%, item consistency (ICC) <0.8 and item variance <1 on an a priori basis (p. 79-80). 42 items (see Appendix B) were removed, producing the working version of the MICE index (MICE-38). The MICE-38 index was assessed again for reliability and validity by performing the previous tests using the MICE-80 data set adjusted for item removal. The reliability coefficient was 0.963 (95% CI 0.944 - 0.977) (p. 85). The MICE-38 index maintained known-groups validity: 15% higher scores in good studies (95% CI 4 - 25, p = 0.006) (p. 89). Correlation with JIF was again poor (Pearson r = 0.271). The convergent construct hypothesis was supported with statistician-assisted studies scoring higher by 13% (95% CI 7 - 20, p = 0.000) (p. 91). Divergent construct hypothesis also remained supported: absolute Pearson correlations <0.2 (p. 91). Hence, the first hypothesis of producing a reliable and valid score for measuring controlled experimental quality in informatics was demonstrated. The MICE index is applicable to computer science and health informatics, thus demonstrating hypothesis 2 and 3.

In support of the hypotheses, an application of the MICE index was shown (see Chapter 5.) A common area of experimentation in informatics was chosen: summative evaluation of clinical decision support tools and systems. A review of 21 studies from 2007 was conducted and showed that experimental quality was moderately high (mean 0.656, median 0.704, 95% CI 0.583 - 0.729). Reviews, such as the one performed, can be used to monitor the quality of empirical research in informatics in a quantitative way. Such reviews have yet to occur in computer science experimentation.

The review data set provided limited, further data against which to assess the choice of validity tests. No known-groups testing occurred because the review sample was not pre-judged. Criterion validity using JIF was again not supported (Spearman rho = −0.167). Statistician assistance appeared to improve MICE-38 scores by 9% (95% CI −5 - 24%, p = 0.177), but this was not significant; the convergent construct hypothesis was unanswered due to insufficient sample size. The divergent construct hypotheses were partially supported: study quality was not related to the number study authors, references or pages (Spearman rho ≤ 0.254). Year of publication was not tested, since all studies were from 2007.

6.2. Contributions of the Research

6.2.1. The MICE Index

The primary contribution of this research is the MICE index (p. 94): a questionnaire for quantifying the degree of quality of human-based informatics experiments. It has demonstrable reliability (p.

85) and validity (p. 89-91) and can be completed in a short amount of time. The MICE index will be useful for computer science and health informatics experimental researchers to plan and write up their studies; they can use the index as a checklist. It will be useful for readers and assessors of experiments to identify good studies from poor. As more and more scientifically based evidence accumulates in the informatics literature, it will be harder to keep up with important empirical studies. This has happened in medicine, with the explosion in evidence-based medicine, and was the impetus for Sackett to advise skipping nonrandomised studies to save the busy clinician's time (254). As more experimental evidence builds in computer science and health informatics, scores like the MICE index might be used to weight results for meta-analysis. For researchers who are monitoring the quality of experimental evidence, the MICE index will be a practical tool.

The MICE index may be ahead of its time in computer science. Experimentation is becoming more and more used as a research method, especially when humans are involved (in developing or using ICT). Advocacy research has had its day (15), just as the self-proclaimed experts in medicine of yesteryear had theirs. Evidence-based computer science and informatics is the emerging future. However, at this point in time, experimentation is too focussed at the level of software engineering, and experimental quality is still at the guideline development stage. With time, as happened for medicine, computer science will need instruments to measure experimental quality. With the influence of medicine, health informatics has already started on this path.

6.2.2.   Improving Methods for Creating Informatics Experimental Quality Scores
One of the difficulties in developing the MICE index was that no suitable yardstick was available to test criterion validity. A simple method for assessing validity is for the new scale and current scale to measure a series of objects and examine the correlation. However, the yardstick should have good psychometric properties to allow a meaningful correlational study. The MICE index could be used in the future as the yardstick for other instruments. In this way, this research has contributed to the psychometric development of future scales.

This research examined the construct of informatics experimental quality in ways that other research has not. While health informatics scales exist, none of them discuss the psychometric appropriateness of their development. This research asked of itself: what is quality (p.32, 60)? Is it homogeneous? What is its level of measurement (p. 34)? How can nominal responses be continuous (p. 119)? In fairness, such exploration may be too long for a journal article that contains a scale and its applied use, but the psychometric principles of informatics scale should be examined somewhere. A glaring omission from the all of the health informatics scales encountered in this research was the lack of formal validity testing. In particular, construct validity testing, the strongest form of validity (138) (p. 132), requires multiple hypothesis tests. To the author's knowledge, this research is the first that provides hypotheses about how experimental quality might behave (effect of statistical assistance and relationship to author/reference/page counts and publication year). While some of these might be problematic (see Limitations of the Research below), this research provides some ground upon which to build. To repeat Streiner and Norman, "Scale constructors are limited only by their imagination in devising experiments to test their hypotheses." (131) (p. 174), but such work must occur.

As part of understanding experimental quality in informatics, MICE scores were assessed for normality. It was found, overall, that scores were near normal (p. 68, 85). This contributes to the knowledge base about the properties of quality. Future work may build upon such a finding. It also has implication for what might be considered "good" and "poor" quality. This research did not explicitly define a MICE score that is "good" or "poor". Such thresholds might be arbitrary and criterion-referenced or, if quality is normal, norm-referenced, e.g. 2 standard deviations away from the mean defines good and poor.

6.2.3. Measurement: a Wider Issue
One of the themes of this research is the importance of measurement. This issue is broader than that of measuring experimental quality. Computer science and health informatics are replete will measurement issues. There are many vague things: software complexity, user friendliness, business process improvement, clinical appropriateness etc. What is the nature of the things that we measure? Can we test for or assume the properties of these things and, if so, how or why? This research emphasised measurement and may stimulate good measurement practice in other areas of informatics.

6.2.4. Experimentation as Science and Foundation for Disciplines
This research has fostered experimentation as an avenue for scientific foundation in computer science and health informatics. In Chapter 1, it was noted that Brooks described computer science as not science but engineering. Some might view health informatics in the same way, i.e. merely the engineering/application of computer-based tools to support health care. There is certainly a place for the construction of computing artefacts in health care and other domains. Important problems in the world have been solved by the creation of tools. However, this does not mean computer science and health informatics are not scientific. Engineering theories allow construction of objects with confidence in predicting their behaviours. However, those theories must somehow still be established. They may be derived mathematically. In informatics, where human involvement adds messiness, theories can be experimentally derived. Engineers, being able to confidently predict that

acceleration is independent of mass, might scoff at the idea of experimentation. They would forget Galileo, who rolled different balls down an incline to investigate it (315). So, when McManus asserted that reliance on randomised controlled trials in medicine shows a failure of confidence in theories, he was not quite correct (118); theory can be established by experimentation. While other research methods and paradigms are important, good quality experimentation can further computer science and health informatics as science.

This research highlighted the difficulties of where research in health informatics should be placed. Experimentation has much to offer computer science and health informatics, and this is recognised by researchers in both areas. However, experimentation has developed in both in isolation from each other. If a controlled experiment is to be used to assess the effectiveness of a computer technology on human outcomes, it seems unwise to develop experimental methods for general computing and ones for health computing. Yet, computer science has not learned from health informatics and vice versa. Indeed, it was noted in the literature review of experimentation in Chapter 3 that health informatics is more closely aligned to medicine than computer science. This research is unique in that it examined experimentation from both fields. Notably, health informatics scales and experimental guidelines make no reference to the computer science literature. It is unfortunate that health informatics only borrows computational methods from computer science but ignores the empirical developments. On the other hand, computer science also does not have to reinvent the wheel when empirical methods have been used in health informatics. Therefore, this research made a small step in the unification of the 2 fields in the context of experimental quality. Without collaboration, it is predicted that both fields will continue to develop evaluation and experimentation in isolation, and this will contribute to the divisions discussed in the first chapter.

6.2.5. Review of Recent Clinical Decision Support Tool Experimental Quality

Chapter 5 presented an application of the MICE index but also produced a small review of experiments in clinical decision support systems. It contributes by being a recent review of a common type of health informatics experiment. It can be built upon by reviewing subsequent years to generate trends in quality and experimental problems for addressing.

6.3. Limitations of the Research

The brainstorming of experimental concepts from literature sources was performed by one judge (the author) (p. 60-62). Concepts that were similar in meaning may not have been as similar to another judge. There was no attempt to measure rater agreement on concept meaning or similarities.

Similarly, the selection of pooled concepts for inclusion into the questionnaire was based on one judge. This may have introduced bias. Another option would have been to use the Delphi method.

Test-retest reliability can be problematic (p. 64). The choice of test-retest reliability was made on pragmatic grounds. Detractors of test-retest reliability criticise it for memory effects, single-rater interpretation of scale items and changes in attribute level between periods of time. Memory effect refers to the scale user remembering how she answered the last time and simply putting it down on the questionnaire again rather than treating the item newly and considering again. It is recommended that the interval between tests consists of 2 to 14 days (131) (p. 137). In this research, the interval was 3 to 4 weeks and beyond the ability of the author to remember the answers to previous items. Each study was read and assessed again as if new, but it is possible that content could have been remembered or better understood with repetition. There is empirical evidence that memory effects are overrated; McKelvie experimentally studied memory effects (using a 3 week test-retest interval) and found they did not greatly increase reliability coefficients (210). Single-rater interpretation of items is a potential problem when assessment scales are developed for various raters to use. Can it be guaranteed that several raters will interpret the written item in the same way? Also, will they answer based on their experience of experimentation in the same way? These sources of error are not detected well by test-retest using a single rater. The last issue of changing attributes is less of a problem for studying experimental quality than, for instance, psychological attributes. While people can change between points in time and, therefore, reflect change in scale scores (completely unrelated to an instrument's reliability), experimental quality is constant. Unless there is a paradigm shift in experimental concepts, studies measured weeks apart will be stable.

The choice of divergent hypothetical constructs was not ideal in retrospect (p. 77). Divergent hypotheses are useful, as they approach a construct from another direction. However, the hypothesis may not actually be divergent in theory. For example, initially it was hypothesised that publication year should not be correlated with experimental quality. It is possible, though, that quality of experiments improves over time; in which case, it would be a convergent hypothesis, and the absence of a correlation would not support the MICE index's validity. Perhaps month of publication would have been a better choice. The same problem could have occurred with number of study authors, i.e. more researchers thinking about an experiment may actually improve quality. These problems are not so much a problem with the MICE index but with understanding the behaviour of experimental quality. As noted in Chapter 2 (p. 48), problems can arise due the instrument, the hypothesis or both.

145

While no weighting scheme was applied, there is inadvertent weighting when items tap similar or hierarchical attributes (131) (p. 105). For example, statistical appropriateness overlaps specific statistical errors, e.g. unit of analysis error. Thus, marking down one also marks down the other and effectively weights the scale towards statistical mistakes. This is not so much a limitation of the MICE index but an issue to be considered when creating scales, especially if there are few items.

The reuse of the MICE-80 data set for the MICE-38 reliability (p. 80) and validity tests (p. 89) ignored a potential problem with interpretation of some items. It was noted in Chapter 2 (p. 42) that the answering of items could sometimes depend on the answering of previous items. Hence, removal of items strictly requires de novo application (to the same or different set of studies) instead of recalculation of scores. While most of the items would not have been affected in this way, a small bias was probably introduced.

While the literature review of experimental guidelines covered a large breadth of readings (p. 53-55), it is probable that not all relevant material was retrieved. There are several factors that can limit comprehensiveness: English language bias, bibliographical database selection and availability of library resources. Furthermore, there is reliance upon the search and relevancy functions of online databases. Nevertheless, a large number of sources contributed to the development of the MICE index.

6.4.   Future Work

This research furthers the scientific basis for health informatics and computer science. Research in these fields should have a good experimental foundation. Researchers can build upon the findings herein to improve:

- The quality of their experimental research.

- The understanding of experimental quality as it relates to human-based informatics experiments.

- The reliability and validity of other measurement instruments developed in the future.

Research into human interaction with informatics methods and artefacts is not limited to controlled experimentation, and there is potential for other forms of empirical methods to be assessed for quality. This research demonstrated the importance of good research methodology and how quality assurance may be delivered. Future work may focus on, for instance, qualitative evaluative methods.

This work will stimulate further discussions about evidence in computing and informatics. With ever-increasing research findings being published, we should be assessing the credibility and usefulness of this evidence. Evidence-based practice is a new area of research in computer science. Quantitative assessment of evidence quality will be the next frontier. Methodological reviews using good instruments should be undertaken by empirical researchers. In health informatics, we should be continuing the assessment of evidence, but we should do so with validated instruments. Further work needs to be done in quantitative meta-analysis of evidence in informatics. Eventually, repositories of high quality informatics evidence could be established in a similar fashion to the Cochrane Collaboration (www.cochrane.org).

This work will also stimulate thinking into how we should avoid unnecessary duplication of efforts in informatics experimentation. If educators are to teach experimental research methods in informatics and computer science, there should be further work to consolidate common ideas applicable to discipline-specific areas of informatics. Also, this research can be used to teach informatics students about experimental principles and get them critically thinking. Further research can examine the best ways to get students to think critically about empirical knowledge.

Future work should also include improving the MICE index. Scale development is iterative. This work began efforts into analysing the properties of experimental quality in computer science and health informatics. More convergent and divergent hypothetical constructs need to be assessed. The MICE index should be tested against other raters and with other experimental studies. If a known-groups approach is used, any expert panel that categorises study quality should itself be reliable enough to discriminate at the desired level. The panel should also be knowledgeable in computer science and health informatics experiments. Similarly, raters applying the MICE index for inter-rater reliability should have experience with computer science and health informatics experiments. Future work might also show that the scale could be shorter without sacrificing its properties. There is also potential for experimental scales to be defined and developed for other areas of informatics.

6.5.   Final Words

Despite the limitations in developing and testing the MICE index, this research has made contributions to computer science and health informatics at a basic science level. When experimentation is done well, it is a powerful tool in the researcher's kit. When good experiments direct the development and use of ICT and information resources, the potential of such tools is closer to being achieved.

References

1.   Lewis T, Smith W. The computer science debate: it's a matter of perspective. ACM SIGCSE Bulletin 2005;37(2):80-4.

2.   Gal-Ezer J, Harel D. What (else) should CS educators know? Communications of the ACM 1998;41(9):77-84.

3.   Parlante N. What is computer science? ACM SIGCSE Bulletin 2005;37(2):24-5.

4.   Denning P, Comer D, Gries D, Mulder M, Tucker A, Turner A, et al. Computing as a discipline. Communications of the ACM 1989;32(1):9-23.

5.   Wulf W. Are we scientists or engineers? ACM Computing Surveys 1995;27(1):55-7.

6.   Abernethy K, Gabbert P, Treu K, Piergari G, Reichgelt H. Impact of the emerging discipline of information technology on computing curricula: some experiences. Journal of Computing Sciences in Colleges 2005;21(2):237-43.

7.   Gregg D, Kulkarni U, Vinze A. Understanding the philosophical underpinnings of software engineering research in information systems. Information Systems Frontiers 2001;3(2):169-83.

8.   Khazanchi D, Munkvold B. Is information systems a science? An inquiry into the nature of the information systems discipline. The DATABASE for Advances in Information Systems 2000;31(3):24-42.

9.   Pather S, Remenyi D. Some of the philosophical issues underpinning research in information systems: from positivism to critical realism. In: Proceedings of SAICSIT 2004; Stellenbosch, South Africa. South African Institute for Computer Scientists and Information Technologists; 2004. p. 141-6.

10.   Mackay W, Fayard A. HCI, natural science and design: a framework for triangulation across disciplines. In: Symposium of Designing Interactive Systems. Proceedings of the Conference on Designing Interactive Systems: Processes, Practices, Methods, and Techniques; Amsterdam, The Netherlands. ACM Press; 1997. p. 223-34.

11.   The Joint Task Force for Computing Curricula. Computing Curricula 2005. New York, USA: Association for Computing Machinery; 2005.

12.   Dijkstra E. On a cultural gap. The Mathematical Intelligencer 1986;8(1):48-52.

13.   Brooks F. The computer scientist as a toolsmith II. Communications of the ACM 1996;39(3):61-8.

14.   Kasanen E, Lukka K, Sittonen A. The constructive approach in management accounting. Journal of Management Accounting Research 1993;5:243-64.

15.   Glass RL. The software-research crisis. Software, IEEE 1994;11(6):42-47.

16.   Fenton N, Pfleeger SL, Glass RL. Science and substance: a challenge to software engineers. Software, IEEE 1994;11(4):86-95.

17.   Brilliant S, Knight J. Empirical research in software engineering: a workshop. ACM SIGSOFT 1999;24(3):44-52.

18.   Tichy W. Should computer scientists experiment more? Computer 1998;31(5):32-40.

19.   Zelkowitz M, Wallace D. Experimental validation in software engineering. Information and Software Technology 1997;39(11):735-43.

20.   Stewart N. Science and computer science. ACM Computing Surveys 1995;27(1):39-41.

21.   Denning P. What is experimental computer science? Communications of the ACM 1980;23(10):543-4.

22.   Loui M. Computer science is a new engineering discipline. ACM Computing Surveys 1995;27(1):31-2.

23.   Widrow B, Hartenstein R, Hecht-Nielsen R. Eulogy [homepage on the Internet]. 2005 [updated cited 7 Mar 2008]. [1 screens]. Available from: http://helios.informatik.uni-kl.de/eulogy.pdf

24.   Fourman M. Informatics. Edinburgh, Scotland: Division of Informatics, The Universtiy of Edinburgh; 2002.

25.   Buerck J, Feig D. Knowledge discovery and dissemination: a curriculum model for informatics. SIGCSE Bulletin 2006;38(4):48-51.

26.   Mohr J. Teaching medical informatics: teaching on the seams of disciplines, cultures, traditions. Methods of Information in Medicine 1989;28:273-80.

27.   Logan J, Price S. Computer science education for medical informaticians. International Journal of Medical Informatics 2004;73(2):139-44.

28.   Blois M. Medical informatics in medical school: should we teach concepts or procedures? ACM SIGBIO Newsletter 1987;9(3):38-41.

29.   Detmer D. Medical informatics: a mutagenic force for artistry and science in the healing professions. Methods of Information in Medicine 1996;35(3):178-80.

30.   Warner H. A view of medical informatics as an academic discipline. Computers and Biomedical Research 1993;26(4).

31.   Hasman A, Haux R, Albert A. A systematic view on medical informatics. Computer Methods and Programs in Biomedicine 1996;51(3):131-9.

32.   International Medical Informatics Association [homepage on the Internet]. Edmonton, Canada: [updated unknown; cited 5 Jul 2008]. [2 screens]. Available from: http://www.imia.org

33.   Haux R. Medical informatics: once more towards systematization. Methods of Information in Medicine 1996;35(3):189-92.

34.   Haux R. On medical informatics. Methods of Information in Medicine 1989;28(2):69-77.

35.   Kay S. Medical informatics: 'making the computer go away'. Proceedings of the Annual International Conference of the IEEE Engineering in Medicine and Biology Society 1991;13(3):1375-77.

36.   Haynes R, Jadad A, Hunt D. What's up in health informatics? Canadian Medical Association Journal 1997;1718-9.

37.   Gremy F. Random reflections on science, technique and art, applied to medicine and medical informatics. Methods of Information in Medicine 1996;35(3):173-7.

38.   Warner H. Medical informatics: a real discipline? Journal of the American Medical Informatics Association 1995;2(4):207-14.

39.   Imhoff M, Webb A, Goldschmidt A. Health informatics. Intensive Care Medicine 2001;27(1):179-86.

40.   De Lusignan S. What is primary care informatics? Journal of the American Medical Informatics Association 2003;10(4):304-9.

41.   Heathfield H, Wyatt J. Medical informatics: hiding our light under a bushel, or the emperor's new clothes? Methods of Information in Medicine 1993;32(2):181-2.

42.   Duncan K, Austing R, Katz S, Pengov R, Pogue R, Wasserman A. Health computing: curriculum for an emerging profession - report of the ACM Curriculum Committee on Health Computing Education. In: ACM 78: Proceedings of the 1978 annual conference. Washington, D.C., USA: ACM; 1978. p. 277-85.

43.   Shannon R, Duncan K. Why a curriculum in health computing? In: Proceedings of the 1978 ACM Annual Conference; Washington, D.C., USA. ACM; 1978. p. 273-6.

44.   Austing R. Computer science in health computing education. ACM SIGBIO Newsletter 1981;5(SI):46-53.

45.   Duncan K. Medical informatics: clinical decision making and beyond. ACM SIGBIO Newsletter 1988;10(2):38-40.

46.   Kane M, Brewer J, Goldman J, Moidu K. Integrating bioinformatics, clinical informatics, and information technology in support of interdisciplinary curriculum development. In: SIGITE'06: Proceedings of the 7th Conference on Information Technology Education; Minneapolis, USA. ACM; 2006.

47.   Hovenga E, Kidd M. Health informatics in Australia. In: Hovenga E, Kidd M, Cesnik B, editors. Health informatics: an overview. South Melbourne, Australia: Churchill Livingstone; 1996.

48.   International Medical Informatics Association [homepage on the Internet]. Edmonton, Canada: [updated unknown; cited 21 Jun 2008]. [5 screens]. Available from: http://www.imia.org/about.lasso

49.   Association for Computing Machinery [homepage on the Internet]. ACM; 2008 [updated unknown; cited 21 Jun 2008]. Special Interest Groups; [9 screens]. Available from: http://www.acm.org/sigs

50.   IEEE Engineering in Medicine and Biology Society [homepage on the Internet]. EMBS; [updated 20 Jun 2008; cited 21 Jun 2008]. [7 screens]. Available from: http://www.embs.org/aboutus.html

51.   Dimitroff A. Medical informatics conference papers: a content analysis of research in a new discipline. Computers and Biomedical Research 1994;27(4):276-90.

52.   JAMIA - Journal of the American Medical Informatics Association [homepage on the Internet]. Hanley & Belfus; 2005 [updated unknown; cited 21 Jun 2008]. [40 screens]. Available from: http://www.jamia.org/misc/ifora.shtml

53.   International Journal of Medical Informatics [homepage on the Internet]. Elsevier; 2007 [updated unknown; cited 21 Jun 2008]. [5 screens]. Available from: http://www.elsevier.com/wps/find/journaldescription.cws_home/506040/authorinstructions

54.   Ammenwerth E, Brender J, Nykanen P, Prokosch H, Rigby M, Talmon J. Visions and strategies to improve evaluation of health information systems: reflections and lessons based on the HIS-EVAL workshop in Innsbruck. International Journal of Medical Informatics 2004;73(6):479-91.

55.   Perry G, Roderer N, Assar S. A current perspective on medical informatics and health sciences librarianship. Journal of the Medical Library Association 2005;93(2):199-205.

56.   Whetton S. Health informatics: who am I (and does it really matter)? In: Westbrook J, Callen J, editors. HIC 2006 Bridging the Digital Divide: Clinician, Consumer and Computer; Sydney, Australia. HISA; 2006.

57.   Shahar Y. Medical informatics: between science and engineering, between academia and industry. Methods of Information in Medicine 2002;41(1):8-11.

58.   Protti D, Van Bemmel J, Gunzenhauser R, Haux R, Warner H, Douglas J, et al. Can health/medical informatics be regarded as a separate discipline? Methods of Information in Medicine 1994;33(3):318-26.

59.   Musen M. Medical informatics: searching for underlying components. Methods of Information in Medicine 2002;41(1):12-9.

60.   Reichertz P. Preparing for change: concepts and education in medical informatics. Computer Methods and Programs in Biomedicine 1987;25(2):89-102.

61.   Wyatt J. Medical informatics: artefacts of science? Methods of Information in Medicine 1996;35(3):197-200.

62.   Smith J, Buerck J. A multidisciplinary approach to graduate education in informatics - a proposal in process. Journal of Computing Sciences in Colleges 2007;22(4):39-45.

63.   Masys D, Flateley Brennan P, Ozbolt J, Corn M, Shortliffe E. Are medical informatics and nursing informatics distinct disciplines? Journal of the American Medical Informatics Association 1999;7(3):304-12.

64.   Leven F, Knaup P, Schmidt D, Wetter T. Medical informatics at Heidelberg/Heilbronn: status—evaluation—new challenges in a specialised curriculum for medical informatics after thirty years of evolution. International Journal of Medical Informatics 2004;73(2):117-25.

65.   Bouman L, Swetsloot-Schonk J, Jaspers M, Louter G, Timmers T. The graduate training in medical information sciences in the Academic Medical Centre at the University of Amsterdam. International Journal of Medical Informatics 1998;50(1-3):151-7.

66.   Heathfield H, Wyatt J. The road to professionalism in medical informatics: a proposal for debate. Methods of Information in Medicine 1995;34(5):426-33.

67.   Johnson S. A framework for the biomedical informatics curriculum. In: AMIA 2003 Symposium Proceedings; Washington, D.C., USA. AMIA; 2003. p. 331-5.

68.   Wyatt JC, Wyatt SM. When and how to evaluate health information systems? International Journal of Medical Informatics 2003;69(2-3):251-59.

69.   Wyatt J, Spiegelhalter D. Evaluating medical expert systems: what to test and how? Medical Informatics 1990;15(3):205-17.

70.   Rector A. Art and science - problems and solutions. Methods of Information in Medicine 1996;35(3):181-4.

71.   Council on Scientific Affairs and Council on Long Range Planning and Development of the American Medical Association. Medical informatics: an emerging medical discipline. Journal of Medical Systems 1990;14(4):161-79.

72.   Sullivan F. What is health informatics? Journal of Health Services Research & Policy 2001;6(4):251-4.

73. Talmon J, Enning J, Castaneda G, Eurlings F, Hoyer D, Nykanen P, et al. The VATAM guidelines. International Journal of Medical Informatics 1999;56(1-3):107-15.

74. Sackett D, Rosenberg W, Gray J, Haynes R, Richardson W. CEBM Centre for Evidence-Based Medicine [homepage on the Internet]. CEBM; 2008 [updated unknown; cited 17 Jun 2008]. What is EBM?; [5 screens]. Available from: http://www.cebm.net/?o=1014

75. Hertzum M, Simonsen J. Evidence-based development: a viable approach? In: Proceedings of the 3rd Nordic Conference on Human-Computer Interaction; Tampere, Finland. ACM Press; 2004. p. 385-8.

76. Kitchenham B, Dyba T, Jorgensen M. Evidence-based software engineering. In: Proceedings of the 26th International Conference on Software Engineering; Washington, D.C., USA. IEEE Computer Society; 2004. p. 273-81.

77. Shortliffe E. Professionalism in medical informatics. Methods of Information in Medicine 1996;35(3):155-6.

78. Tierney W, Overhage J, McDonald C. A plea for controlled trials in medical informatics. Journal of the American Medical Informatics Association 1994;1(4):353-5.

79. Tan K, Dear P, Newell S. Clinical decision support systems for neonatal care. The Cochrane Database of Systematic Reviews 2005 2005(2):1-18.

80. Moher T, Schneider G. Methodology and experimental research in software engineering. International Journal of Man-Machine Studies 1982;16:65-87.

81. Talmon J, Hasman A. Medical informatics as a discipline at the beginning of the 21st century. Methods of Information in Medicine 2002;41(1):4-7.

82. Shortliffe E, Cimino J. Biomedical informatics: computer applications in health care and biomedicine. 3rd ed. New York, USA: Springer Science+Business Media; 2006.

83. Huang Q. Competencies for graduate curricula in health, medical and biomedical informatics: a framework. Health Informatics Journal 2007;13(2):89-103.

84. Maojo V, Kulikowski C. Medical informatics and bioinformatics: integration or evolution through scientific crises? Methods of Information in Medicine 2006;45(5):474-82.

85. Dube L, Pare G. Rigor in information systems positivist case research: current practices, trends, and recommendations. MIS Quarterly 2003;27(4):597-635.

86. Klecun E, Cornford T. A critical approach to evaluation. European Journal of Information Systems 2005;14:229-43.

87. Harrison R, Badoo N, Barry E, Biffl S, Parra A, Winter B, et al. Directions and methodologies for empirical software engineering research. Empirical Software Engineering 1999;4(4):405-10.

88. Perry D, Porter A, Votta L. Empirical studies of software engineering: a roadmap. In: Proceedings of the Conference on The Future of Software Engineering; Limerick, Ireland. ACM Press; 2000. p. 345-55.

89. Holloway C. Software engineering and epistemology. ACM SIGSOFT 1995;20(2):20-1.

90. Tichy W, Lukowicz P, Prechelt L, Heinz E. Experimental evaluation in computer science: a quantitative study. Journal of Systems and Software 1995;28(1):9-18.

91.   Sjoberg D, Hannay J, Hansen O, Kampenes V, Karahasanovic A, Liborg N, et al. A survey of controlled experiments in software engineering. IEEE Transactions on Software Engineering 2005;31(9):733-52.

92.   Basili V. The role of experimentation in software engineering: past, current and future. In: Proceedings of the 18th International Conference on Software Engineering; Berlin, Germany. IEEE Computer Society; 1996.

93.   Kitchenham B, Budgen D, Brereton P, Linkman S. Realising evidence-based software engineering. In: International Conference on Software Engineering. Proceedings of the 2005 Workshop on Realising Evidence-Based Software Engineering; St Louis, Missouri, USA. ACM Press; 2005. p. 1-3.

94.   Sjoberg D, Anda B, Arisholm E, Dyba T, Jorgensen M, Karahasanovic A, et al. Conducting realistic experiments in software engineering. In: Proceedings of the 2002 International Symposium on Empirical Software Engineering.; Nara, Japan. IEEE Computer Society; 2002.

95.   Wade M, Tingling P. A new twist on an old method: a guide to the applicability and use of web experiments in information systems research. The DATABASE for Advances in Information Systems 2005;36(3):69-88.

96.   Braught G, Miller C, Reed D. Core empirical concepts and skills for computer science. In: Proceedings of the 35th SIGCSE Technical Symposium on Computer Science Education; Norfolk, Virginia, USA. ACM Press; 2004. p. 245-9.

97.   Fenwick J, Norris C, Wilkes J. Scientific experimentation via the matching game. In: Proceedings of the 33rd SIGCSE Technical Symposium on Computer Science Education; Cincinnati, Kentucky. ACM Press; 2002. p. 326-30.

98.   Chuang J, Hripcsak G, Heitjan D. Design and analysis of controlled trials in naturally clustered environments. Journal of the American Medical Informatics Association 2002;9(3):230-8.

99.   Wyatt J. Quantitative evaluation of clinical software, exemplified by decision support systems. International Journal of Medical Informatics 1997;47(3):165-73.

100.   Moher T, Schneider G. Methods for improving controlled experimentation in software engineering. In: Proceedings of the 5th International Conference on Software Engineering; San Diego, California, USA. IEEE Press; 1981. p. 224-33.

101.   Zannier C, Melnik G, Maurer F. On the success of empirical studies in the International Conference on Software Engineering. In: Proceedings of the 28th International Conference on Software Engineering; Shanghai, China. ACM Press; 2006. p. 341-50.

102.   Tichy W. Hints for reviewing empirical work in software engineering. Empirical Software Engineering 2000;5(4):309-12.

103.   National Health and Medical Research Council. How to use the evidence: assessment and application of scientific evidence. Canberra, Australia: National Health and Medical Research Council; 2000.

104.   Wikipedia, the free encyclopedia [homepage on the Internet]. 2008 [updated 5 Jun 2008; cited 11 Jun 2008]. Evidence-based medicine; [11 screens]. Available from: http://en.wikipedia.org/wiki/Evidence-based_medicine

105.   Chan S, Bhandari M. The quality of reporting of orthopaedic randomized trials with use of a checklist for nonpharmacological therapies. The Journal of Bone and Joint Surgery, American Volume 2007;89(9):1970-8.

106.   Farrokhyar F, Chu R, Whitlock R, Thabane L. A systematic review of the quality of publications reporting coronary artery bypass grafting trials. Canadian Journal of Surgery 2007;50(4):266-77.

107.   Hill C, Buchbinder R, Osborne R. Quality of reporting of randomized clinical trials in abstracts of the 2005 Annual Meeting of the American College of Rheumatology. The Journal of Rheumatology 2007;Epub ahead of print.

108.   Altman D, Schulz K, Moher D, Egger M, Davidoff F, Elbourne D, et al. The revised CONSORT statement for reporting randomized trials: explanation and elaboration. Annals of Internal Medicine 2001;134:663-94.

109.   Moher D, Jadad A, Nichol G, Penman M, Tugwell P, Walsh S. Assessing the quality of randomized controlled trials: an annotated bibliography of scales and checklists. Controlled Clinical Trials 1995;16(62-73).

110.   Verhagen A, De Vet H, De Bie R, Boers M, van den Brandt P. The art of quality assessment of RCTs included in systematic reviews. Journal of Clinical Epidemiology 2001;54:651-4.

111.   Moher D, Jones A, Lepage L. Use of the CONSORT statement and quality of reports of randomized trials. JAMA 2001;285(15):1992-5.

112.   Garg A, Adhikari N, McDonald H, Rosas-Arellano M, Devereaux P, Beyene J, et al. Effects of computerized clinical decision support systems on practitioner performance and patient outcomes: a systematic review. JAMA 2005;293(10):1223-38.

113.   Jedlitschka A, Pfahl D. Reporting guidelines for controlled experiments in software engineering. In: 2005 International Symposium on Empirical Software Engineering; Noosa Heads, Australia. IEEE; 2005. p. 95-104.

114.   Singer J. Using the American Psychological Association (APA) style guidelines to report experimental results. In: Proceedings of the Workshop on Empirical Studies in Software Maintenance; Oxford, England; 1999. p. 71-5.

115.   Moehr J, Anglin C, Schaafsma J, Pantazi S, Grimm N. Lest formalisms impede insight and success: evaluation in health informatics. Methods of Information in Medicine 2006;45:67-72.

116.   Moehr JR. Evaluation: salvation or nemesis of medical informatics? Computers in Biology and Medicine 2002;32(3):113-25.

117.   Kaplan B. Evaluating informatics applications—some alternative approaches: theory, social interactionism, and call for methodological pluralism. International Journal of Medical Informatics 2001;64(1):39-56.

118.   McManus C. Engineering quality in health care. Quality in Health Care 1996;5:127.

119.   Weinberg G. How can we study programming? In: The psychology of computer programming. Silver anniversary ed. New York, USA: Dorset House; 1998.

120.   Weinberg G. Goals and performance in computer programming. Human Factors 1974;16(1):70-7.

121.   Spearman C. The proof and measurement of association between two things. American Journal of Psychology 1904;3:1-18.

122.   Kitchenham B, Pfleeger SL, Hoaglin D, El Emam K, Rosenberg J. Preliminary guidelines for empirical research in software engineering. IEEE Transactions on Software Engineering 2002;28(8):721-34.

123.   Sadler C, Kitchenham B. Evaluating software engineering methods and tool. Part 4: the influence of human factors. ACM SIGSOFT 1996;21(5):11-13.

124.   Pirsig R. Zen and the art of motorcycle maintenance: an inquiry into values. London: Vintage; 1999.

125.   DeVellis R. Scale development: theory and applications. 2nd ed. Thousand Oaks, California, USA: Sage Publications; 2003.

126.   Stevens S. On the theory of scales of measurement. Science 1946;103(2684):677-80.

127.   Gaito J. Measurement scales and statistics: resurgence of an old misconception. Psychological Bulletin 1980;87(3):564-7.

128.   Townsend J, Ashby F. Measurement scales and statistics: the misconception misconceived. Psychological Bulletin 1984;96(2):394-401.

129.   Neisser U, Boodoo G, Bouchard T, Boykin A, Brody N, Ceci S, et al. Intelligence: knowns and unknowns. American Psychologist 1996;51(2):77-101.

130.   Lord F. On the statistical treatment of football numbers. American Psychologist 1953;8(12):750-1.

131.   Streiner D, Norman G. Health measurement scales: a practical guide to their development and use. 3rd ed. New York, USA: Oxford University Press; 2003.

132.   Lui K. Preliminary results for a scale that measures the quality of controlled experiments in computing and health informatics. In: Proceedings of the 2nd International Doctoral Symposium on Empirical Software Engineering. IDoESE 2007; Madrid, Spain. Universidad Politecnica de Madrid; 2007. p. 52-9.

133.   Australian Bureau of Statistics. A guide to the Consumer Price Index 15th series. Canberra, Australia: Commwealth of Australia; 2005.

134.   Streiner D. Being inconsistent about consistency: when coeffcient alpha does and does not matter. Journal of Personality Assessment 2003;80(3):217-22.

135.   de Keizer N, Ammenwerth E. The quality of evidence in health informatics: how did the quality of healthcare IT evaluation publications develop from 1982 to 2005? . International Journal of Medical Informatics 2007;Article in Press, Corrected Proof.

136.   Kline T. Psychological testing: a practical approach to design and evaluation. Thousand Oaks, USA: Sage; 2005.

137.   DeVellis R. Classical test theory. Medical Care 2006;44(11 Suppl 3):S50-9.

138.   Friedman C, Wyatt J. Evaluation methods in biomedical informatics. 2nd ed. New York: Springer; 2006.

139.   Shavelson R, Webb N, Rowley G. Generalizability theory. American Psychologist 1989;44(6):922-32.

140.   Cronbach L, Gleser G, Nanda H, Rajaratnam N. The dependability of behavioral measurements: theory of generalizability for scores and profiles. New York, USA: Wiley; 1972.

141.   Jadad A, Moore A, Carroll D, Jenkinson C, Reynolds D, Gavaghan D, et al. Assessing the quality of reports of randomized clinical trials: is blinding necessary? Controlled Clinical Trials 1996;17:1-12.

142.   Chalmers T, Smith H, Blackburn B, Silverman B, Schroeder B, Reitman D, et al. A method for assessing the quality of a randomized control trial. Controlled Clinical Trials 1981;2:31-49.

143.   Goodman S, Berlin J, Fletcher S, Fletcher R. Manuscript quality before and after peer review and editing at Annals of Internal Medicine. Annals of Internal Medicine 1994;121:11-21.

144.   Miller G. The magical number seven, plus or minus two: some limits on our capacity for processing information. The Psychological Review 1956;63:81-97.

145.   Schwarz N, Knauper B, Hippler H, Noelle-Neumann E, Clark I. Rating scales: numeric values may change the meaning of scale labels. Public Opinion Quarterly 1991;55:570-82.

146.   Balas E, Austin S, Ewigman B, Brown G, Mitchell J. Methods of randomized controlled clinical trials in health services research. Medical Care 1995;33(7):687-99.

147.   Nunnally J. Psychometric theory. 2nd ed. New York, USA: McGraw-Hill; 1978.

148.   Shrout P, Fleiss J. Intraclass correlations: uses in assessing rater reliability. Psychological Bulletin 1979;85(2):620-8.

149.   Cronbach L. Coefficient alpha and the internal structure of tests. Psychometrika 1951;16(3):297-334.

150.   van der Loo R. Overview of published assessment and evaluation studies. In: van Gennip E, Talmon J, editors. Assessment and evaluation of information technologies in medicine. Amsterdam: IOS Press; 1995. p. 261-82.

151.   Harden R, Gleeson F. Assessment of clinical experience using an objective structured clinical examination (OSCE). Medical Education 1979;13:41-54.

152.   Juristo N, Moreno A. Basics of software engineering experimentation. Norwell, Massachussets, USA: Kluwer Academic Publishers; 2001.

153.   Wohlin C, Runeson P, Host M, Ohlsson M, Regnell B, Wesslen A. Experimentation in software engineering: an introduction. Norwell, Massachusetts, USA: Kluwer Academic Publishers; 2000.

154.   de Keizer N, Ammenwerth E. The effects and quality of medical IT evaluation studies: trends in 1982-2002. In: Friedman C, editor. AMIA 2005 Annual Symposium Proceedings. AMIA; 2005. p. 186-90.

155.   Henneckens C, Buring E. Epidemiology in medicine. Boston, Massachussets, USA: Little, Brown and Company; 1987.

156.   Myrtveit I, Stensrud E. A controlled experiment to assess the benefits of estimating with analogy and regression models. IEEE Transactions on Software Engineering 1999;25(4):510-25.

157.   Briand L, Bunse C, Daly J. A controlled experiment for evaluating quality guidelines on the maintainability of object-oriented designs. IEEE Transactions on Software Engineering 2001;27(6):513-30.

158.   Basili V, Selby R, Hutchens D. Experimentation in software engineering. IEEE Transactions on Software Engineering 1986;12(7):733-43.

159.   Basili V, Shull F, Lanubile F. Building knowledge through families of experiments. IEEE Transactions on Software Engineering 1999;25(4):456-73.

160.   Boudreau M, Gefen D, Straub D. Validation in information systems research: a state of the art assessment. MIS Quarterly 2001;25(1):1-16.

161.   Brooks R. Studying programmer behavior experimentally: the problems of proper methodology. Communications of the ACM 1980;23(4):207-13.

162.   Host M, Wohlin C, Thelin T. Experimental context classification: incentives and experience of subjects. In: 27th International Conference on Software Engineering; St. Louis, Missouri. ACM; 2005. p. 470-8.

163.   Jarvenpaa S, Dickson G, DeSanctis G. Methodological issues in experimental IS research: experiences and recommendations. MIS Quarterly 1985;9(2):141-56.

164.   Juristo N, Moreno A, Vegas S. Towards building a solid empirical body of knowledge in testing techniques. ACM SIGSOFT Software Engineering Notes 2004;29(5):1-4.

165.   Kitchenham B, Al-Khilidar H, Ali Babar M, Berry M, Cox K, Keung J, et al. Evaluating guidelines for empirical software engineering studies. In: International Symposium on Empirical Software Engineering '06; Rio de Janeiro, Brazil. ACM; 2006. p. 38-47.

166.   Lott C, Rombach H. Repeatable software engineering experiments for comparing defect-detection techniques. Empirical Software Engineering 1996;1(3):241-77.

167.   Pfleeger S. Experimental design and analysis in software engineering. Part 2: how to set up an experiment. ACM SIGSOFT 1995;20(1):22-6.

168.   Pfleeger S. Experimental design and analysis in software engineering. Part 3: types of experimental design. ACM SIGSOFT 1995;20(2):14-6.

169.   Pfleeger S. Experimental design and analysis in software engineering. Part 4: choosing an experimental design. ACM SIGSOFT 1995;20(3):13-5.

170.   Pfleeger S. Experimental design and analysis in software engineering. Part 5: analyzing the data. ACM SIGSOFT 1995;20(5):14-7.

171.   Johnston M, Langton K, Haynes R, Mathieu A. Effects of computer-based clinical decision support systems on clinician performance and patient outcome. Annals of Internal Medicine 1994;120(2):135-42.

172.   Chalmers I, Adams M, Dickersin K, Hetherington J, Tarnow-Mordi W, Meinert C, et al. A cohort study of summary reports of controlled trials. JAMA 1990;263(10):1401-5.

173.   Cho M, Bero L. Instruments for assessing the quality of drug studies published in the medical literature. JAMA 1994;272(2):101-4.

174.   Colditz G, Miller J, Mosteller F. How study design affects outcomes in comparisons of therapy. I: medical. Statistics in Medicine 1989;8(4):441-54.

175.   Detsky A, Naylor C, O'Rourke K, McGeer A, L'Abbe K. Incorporating variations in the quality of individual randomized trials into meta-analysis. Journal of Clinical Epidemiology 1992;45(3):255-65.

176.   Evans M, Pollock A. A score system for evaluating random control clinical trials of prophylaxis of abdominal surgical wound infection. British Journal of Surgery 1985;72:256-60.

177.   Imperiale T, McCullough A. Do corticosteroids reduce mortality from alcoholic hepatitis? Annals of Internal Medicine 1990;113:299-307.

178.   Kleijnen J, Knipschild P, ter Riet G. Clinical trials of homeopathy. BMJ 1991;302:316-23.

179.   Reisch J, Tyson J, Mize S. Aid to the evaluation of therapeutic studies. Pediatrics 1989;84(5):815-27.

180.   Verhagen A, de Vet H, de Bie R, Kessels A, Boers M, Bouter L, et al. The Delphi list: a criteria list for quality assessment of randomized clinical trials for conducting systematic reviews developed by Delphi consensus. Journal of Clinical Epidemiology 1998;51(12):1235-41.

181.   Cohen J. A coefficient of agreement for nominal scales. Educational and Psychological Measurement 1960;20(1):37-46.

182.   Sirkin R. Statistics for the social sciences. Thousand Oaks, California, USA: Sage Publications; 1995.

183.   Hunt D, Haynes R, Hanna S, Smith K. Effects of computer-based clinical decision support systems on physician performance and patient outcomes: a systematic review. JAMA 1998;280(15):1339-46.

184.   de Keizer N, Ammenwerth E. The quality of evidence in health informatics: how did the quality of healthcare IT evaluation publications develop from 1982 to 2005? . International Journal of Medical Informatics 2007;doi:10.1016/j.ijmedinf.2006.11.009.

185.   Diekhoff G. Statistics for the social and behavioral sciences: univariate, bivariate, multivariate. Dubuque, USA: Wm C Brown Publishers; 1992.

186.   Harris M. Basic statistics for behavioral science research. Needham Heights, Massachusetts, USA: Allyn & Bacon; 1995.

187.   Ali Babar M, Biffl S. Eliciting better quality architecture evaluation scenarios: a controlled experiment on top-down vs. bottom-up. In: Proceedings of the 2006 ACM/IEEE International Symposium on Empirical Software Engineering ISESE06; Rio de Janeiro, Brazil. ACM; 2006. p. 307-15.

188.   Ali Babar M, Kitchenham B, Jeffery R. Distributed versus face-to-face meetings for architecture evaluation: a controlled experiment. In: Proceedings of the 2006 ACM/IEEE International Symposium on Empirical Software Engineering ISESE06; Rio de Janeiro, Brazil. ACM; 2006.

189.   Anda B, Sjoberg D. Applying use cases to design versus validate class diagrams – a controlled experiment using a professional modelling tool. In: Proceedings of the 2003 International Symposium on Empirical Software Engineering (ISESE'03). IEEE Computer Society; 2003. p. 50.

190.   Arisholm E, Sjoberg D, Jorgensen M. Assessing the changeability of two object-oriented design alternatives - a controlled experiment. Empirical Software Engineering 2001;6(3):231-77.

191.   Bunse C. Using patterns for the refinement and translation of UML models: a controlled experiment. Empirical Software Engineering 2006;11(2):227-67.

192.   Canfora G, Cimitile A, Garcia F, Piattini M, Vissagio C. Evaluating advantages of test driven development: a controlled experiment with professionals. In: Proceedings of the 2006 ACM/IEEE International Symposium on Empirical Software Engineering ISESE06; Rio de Janeiro, Brazil. ACM; 2006. p. 364-71.

193.   Golden E, John B, Bass L. The value of a usability-supporting architectural pattern in software architecture design: a controlled experiment. In: Proceedings of the 27th International Conference on Software Engineering ICSE '05; St Louis, USA. ACM; 2005. p. 460-9.

194.   Hu P, Zhang Z, Chan W, Tse T. An empirical comparison between direct and indirect test result checking approaches. In: Proceedings of the Third International Workshop on Software Quality Assurance (SOQUA'06); Portland, USA. ACM; 2006. p. 6-13.

195.   Johnson P, Tjahjono D. Assessing software review meetings: a controlled experiment study using CSRS. In: Proceedings of the 19th International Conference on Software Engineering ICSE '97; Boston, USA; 1997. p. 118-27.

196.   Lopes A, Feldman M, Heller R. A controlled experiment with software for teaching Ada tasking. In: Proceedings of the Conference on TRI-Ada '93; Seattle, USA. ACM; 1993. p. 116-25.

197.   Lott C. A controlled experiment to evaluate on-line process guidance. Empirical Software Engineering 1997;2(3):269-89.

198.   Muller M. Two controlled experiments concerning the comparison of pair programming to peer review. The Journal of Systems and Software 2005;78(2):166-79.

199.   Myers G. A controlled experiment in program testing and code walkthroughs/inspections. Communications of the ACM 1978;21(9):760-8.

200.   Ng T, Cheung S, Chan W, Yu Y. Work experience versus refactoring to design patterns: a controlled experiment. In: Proceedings of the 14th ACM SIGSOFT International Symposium on Foundations of Software Engineering SIGSOFT '06/FSE-14; Portland, USA. ACM; 2006. p. 12-22.

201.   Prechelt L, Tichy W. A controlled experiment to assess the benefits of procedure argument type checking. IEEE Transactions on Software Engineering 1998;24(4):302-12.

202.   Prechelt L, Unger B, Tichy W, Votta L. A controlled experiment in maintenance comparing design patterns to simpler solutions. IEEE Transactions on Software Engineering 2001;27(12):1134-44.

203.   Prechelt L, Unger-Lamprecht B, Philippsen M, Tichy W. Two controlled experiments assessing the usefulness of design pattern documentation in program maintenance. IEEE Transactions on Software Engineering 2002;28(6):595-606.

204.   Prechelt L, Unger B, Philippsen M, Tichy W. A controlled experiment on inheritance depth as a cost factor for code maintenance. The Journal of Systems and Software 2003;65(2):115-26.

205.   Sears A, Schneiderman B. Split menus: effectively using selection frequency to organize menus. ACM Transactions on Computer-Human Interaction 1994;1(1):27-51.

206.   Sonnenwald D, Whitton M, Maglaughlin K. Evaluating a scientific collaboratory: results of a controlled experiment. ACM Transactions on Computer-Human Interaction 2003;10(2):150-76.

207.   Vokac M, Tichy W, Sjoberg D, Arisholm E, Aldrin M. A controlled experiment comparing the maintainability of programs designed with and without design patterns - a replication in a real programming environment. Empirical Software Engineering 2004;9(3):149-95.

208.   Wojcicki M, Strooper P. Maximising the information gained from an experimental analysis of code inspection and static analysis for concurrent java components. In: Proceedings of the 2006 ACM/IEEE International Symposium on Empirical Software Engineering ISESE06; Rio de Janeiro, Brazil. ACM; 2006. p. 174-83.

209.   Zettel J. Methodology support in CASE tools and its impact on individual acceptance and use: a controlled experiment. Empirical Software Engineering 2005;10(3):367-94.

210.   McKelvie S. Does memory contaminate test-retest reliability? Journal of General Psychology 1992;119(1):59-72.

211.   Garson G. PA765 Quantitative Research in Public Administration [homepage on the Internet]. NC State University; 2006 [updated 2006; cited 3 November 2006]. PA 765: Reliability Analysis; [13 screens]. Available from: http://www2.chass.ncsu.edu/garson/pa765/reliab.htm

212.	Bonevski B, Sanson-Fisher R, Campbell E, Carruthers A, Reid A, Ireland M. Randomized controlled trial of a computer strategy to increase general practitioner preventive care. Preventive Medicine 1999;29(6):478-86.

213.	Brownbridge G, Evans A, Fitter M, Platts M. An interactive computerized protocol for the management of hypertension: effects on general practitioner's clinical behaviour. Journal of the Royal College of General Practitioners 1986;36(286):198-202.

214.	Cannon D, Allen S. A comparison of the effects of computer and manual reminders on compliance with a mental health clinical practice guideline. Journal of the American Medical Informatics Association 2000;7(2):196-203.

215.	Christakis D, Zimmerman F, Wright J, Garrison M, Rivara F, Davis R. A randomized controlled trial of point-of-care evidence to improve the antibiotic prescribing practices for otitis media in children. Pediatrics 2001;107(2):e15.

216.	Demakis J, Beauchamp C, Cull W, Denwood R, Eisen S, Lofgren R, et al. Improving resident's compliance with standards of ambulatory care: results from the VA Cooperative Study on computerized reminders. JAMA 2000;284(11):1411-16.

217.	Dexter P, Wolinsky F, Gramelspacher G, Zhou X, Eckert G, Waisburd M, et al. Effectiveness of computer-generated reminders for increasing discussions about advance directives and completion of advance directive forms: a randomized controlled trial. Annals of Internal Medicine 1998;128(2):102-10.

218.	Fitzmaurice D, Hobbs F, Murray E, Bradley C, Holder R. Evaluation of computerized decision support for oral anticoagulation management based in primary care. British Journal of General Practice 1996;46(410):533-5.

219.	Fitzmaurice D, Hobbs F, Murray E, Holder R, Allan T, Rose P. Oral anticoagulation management in primary care with the use of computerized decision support and near-patient testing. Archives of Internal Medicine 2000;160(15):2343-8.

220.	Gonzalez E, Vanderheyden B, Ornato J, Comstock T. Computer-assisted optimization of aminophylline therapy in the emergency department. American Journal of Emergency Medicine 1989;7(4):395-401.

221.	Hickling K, Begg E, Moore M. A prospective randomised trial comparing individualised pharmacokinetic dosage prediction for aminoglycosides with prediction based on estimated creatinine clearance in critically ill patients. Intensive Care Medicine 1989;15(4):233-7.

222.	Horn W, Popow C, Miksch S, Kirchner L, Seyfang A. Development and evaluation of VIE-PNN, a knowledge-based system for calculating the parenteral nutrition of newborn infants. Artificial Intelligence in Medicine 2002;24(3):217-28.

223.	Kuperman G, Teich J, Tanasijevic M, Ma'Luf N, Rittenberg E, Jha A, et al. Improving response to critical laboratory results with automation: results of a randomized controlled trial. Journal of the American Medical Informatics Association 1999;6(6):512-22.

224.	Lewis G, Sharp D, Bartholomew J, Pelosi A. Computerized assessment of common mental disorders in primary care: effect on clinical outcome. Family Practice 1996;13(2):120-6.

225.	Lowensteyn I, Joseph L, Levinton C, Abrahamowicz M, Steinert Y, Grover S. Can computerized risk profiles help patients improve their coronary risk? The results of the Coronary Health Assessment Study (CHAS). Preventive Medicine 1998;27(5):730-7.

226.	Mazzuca S, Vinicor F, Einterz R, Tierney W, Norton J, Kalasinki L. Effects of the clinical environment on physicians' response to postgraduate medical education. American Educational Research Journal 1990;27(3):473-88.

161

227. McAlister N, Covvey H, Tong C, Lee A, Wigle E. Randomised controlled trial of computer assisted management of hypertension in primary care. BMJ 1986;293(6548):670-4.

228. McDonald C, Hui S, Smith D, Tierney W, Cohen S, Weinberger M, et al. Reminders to physicians from an introspective computer medical record: a two year randomized trial. Annals of Internal Medicine 1984;100(1):130-8.

229. Poller L, Shiach C, MacCallum P, Johansen A, Munster A, Magalhaes A, et al. Multicentre randomised study of computerised anticoagulant dosage. The Lancet 1998;352(9139):1505-9.

230. Rosser W, McDowell I, Newell C. Use of reminders for preventive procedures in family medicine. Canadian Medical Association Journal 1991;145(7):807-14.

231. Rossi R, Every N. A computerized intervention to decrease the use of calcium channel blockers in hypertension. Journal of General Internal Medicine 1997;12(11):672-8.

232. Rotman B, Sullivan A, McDonald T, Brown B, DeSmedt P, Goodnature D, et al. A randomized controlled trial of a computer-based physician workstation in and outpatient setting: implementation barriers to outcome evaluation. Journal of the American Medical Informatics Association 1996;3(5):340-8.

233. Ryff-de Leche A, Engler H, Nutzi E, Berger M, Berger W. Clinical application of two computerized diabetes management systems: comparison with the log-book method. Diabetes Research 1992;19(3):97-105.

234. Schriger D, Gibbons P, Langone C, Lee S, Altshuler L. Enabling the diagnosis of occult psychiatric illness in the emergency department: a randomized, controlled trial of the computerized, self-administered PRIME-MD diagnostic system. Annals of Emergency Medicine 2001;37(2):132-40.

235. Selker H, Beshansky J, Griffith J, Aufderheide T, Ballin D, Bernard S, et al. Use of the Acute Cardiac Ischemia Time-Insensitive Predictive Insrtument (ACI-TIPI) to assist with triage of patients with chest pain or other symptoms suggestive of acute cardiac ischemia: a multicenter, controlled clinical trial. Annals of Internal Medicine 1998;129(11):845-55.

236. Tamblyn R, Huang A, Perreault R, Jacques A, Roy D, Hanley J, et al. The medical office of the 21st century (MOXXI): effectiveness of computerized decision-making support in reducing inappropriate prescribing in primary care. Canadian Medical Association Journal 2003;169(6):649-56.

237. Tang P, LaRosa M, Newcomb C, Gorden S. Measuring the effects of reminders for outpatient influenza immunizations at the point of clinical opportunity. Journal of the American Medical Informatics Association 1999;6(2):115-21.

238. Thomas J, Moore A, Qualls P. The effect on cost of medical care treated with an automated clinical audit system for patients. Journal of Medical Systems 1983;7(3):307-13.

239. Tierney W, Miller M, Overhage J, McDonald C. Physician inpatient order writing on microcomputer workstations: effects on resource utilization. JAMA 1993;269(3):379-83.

240. Vadher B, Patterson D, Leaning M. Evaluation of a decision support system for initiation and control of oral anticoagulation in a randomised trial. BMJ 1997;314(7089):1252-6.

241. Vadher B, Patterson D, Leaning M. Comparison of oral anticoagulant control by a nurse-practitioner using a computer decision-support system with that by clinicians. Clinical and Laboratory Haematology 1997;19(3):203-7.

242. Verner D, Seligmann H, Platt S, Dany S, Almog S, Zulty L, et al. Computer assisted design of a theophylline dosing regimen in acute bronchospasm: serum concentrations and clinical outcome. European Journal of Clinical Pharmacology 1992;43(1):29-33.

243.   Wexler J, Swender P, Tunnessen W, Orski F. Impact of a system of computer-assisted diagnosis: initial evaluation of the hospitalized patient. American Journal of Diseases of Children 1975;129(2):203-5.

244.   Young D. Improving the consistency with which investigations are requested. Medical Informatics 1981;6(1):13-7.

245.   Moore D, McCabe G. Introduction to the practice of statistics. New York, USA: WH Freeman and Company; 2006.

246.   Garfield E. The history and meaning of the journal impact factor. JAMA 2006;295(1):90-3.

247.   Ha T, Tan S, Soo K. The journal impact factor: too much of an impact? Annals of the Academy of Medicine, Singapore 2006;35(12):911-6.

248.   Saha S. Impact factor: a valid measure of journal quality? Journal of the Medical Library Association 2003;91(1):42-6.

249.   Bath F, Owen V, Bath P. Quality of full and final publications reporting acute stroke trials: a systematic review. Stroke 1998;29(10):2203-10.

250.   Gluud L, Sorensen T, Gotzsche P, Gluud C. The journal impact factor as a predictor of trial quality and outcomes: cohort study of hepatobiliary randomized clinical trials. American Journal of Gastroenterology 2005;100(11):2431-5.

251.   Garfield E. Journal impact factor: a brief review. Canadian Medical Association Journal 1999;161(8):979-80.

252.   World Medical Association General Assembly. World Medical Association Declaration of Helsinki: ethical principles for medical research involving human subjects (revised October 7, 2000). HIV Clinical Trials 2001;2(1):92-5.

253.   Whiting-O'Keefe Q, Henke C, Simbord D. Choosing the correct unit of analysis in Medical Care experiments. Medical Care 1984;22(12):1101-14.

254.   Sackett D. How to read clinical journals: V: to distinguish useful from useless or even harmful therapy. Canadian Medical Association Journal 1981;124(9):1156-62.

255.   Schulz K, Chalmers I, Hayes R, Altman D. Empirical evidence of bias: dimensions of methodological quality associated with estimates of treatment effects in controlled trials. JAMA 1995;273(5):408-12.

256.   Doll W, Deng X, Raghunathan T, Torkzadeh G, Xia W. The meaning and measurement of user satisfaction: a multigroup invariance analysis of the end-user computing satisfaction instrument. Journal of Management Information Systems 2004;21(1):227-62.

257.   Wang A. Information security models and metrics. In: Proceedings of the 43rd Annual Southeast Regional Conference - Volume 2; Kennesaw, USA. ACM; 2005.

258.   Baer R, Dietrich M. Validation of IT-security measurement tools. In: The First International Conference on Availability, Reliability and Security, 2006. ARES 2006; Vienna, Austria. IEEE Computer Society; 2006. p. 980-1.

259.   Cunningham S, Deere S, Symon A, Elton R, McIntosh N. A randomized, controlled trial of computerized physiologic trend monitoring in an intensive care unit. Critical Care Medicine 1998;26(12):2053-60.

260.   Alberdi E, Gilhooly K, Hunter J, Logie R, Lyon A, McIntosh N, et al. Computerisation and decision making in neonatal intensive care: a cognitive engineering investigation. Journal of Clinical Monitoring and Computing 2000;16(2):85-94.

261.   Sibbald B, Roberts C. Understanding controlled trials crossover trials. BMJ 1998;316(7146):1719-20.

262.   Alderson P, Green S. The Cochrane Collaboration open learning material for reviewers [homepage on the Internet]. The Cochrane Collaboration; 2002 [updated Nov 2002; cited 4 Aug 2007]. Issues related to the unit of analysis crossover trials; [2 screens]. Available from: http://www.cochrane-net.org/openlearning/HTML/modA2-3.htm

263.   Eldredge J. The randomised controlled trial design: unrecognized opportunities for health sciences librarianship. Health Information and Libraries Journal 2003;20(s1):34-44.

264.   Rosenthal R, Rubin D. Interpersonal expectancy effects: the first 345 studies. The Behavioral and Brain Sciences 1978;3:377-415.

265.   Noseworthy J, Ebers G, Vandervoot M, Farquhar R, Yetsir E, Roberts R. The impact of blinding on the results of a randomized, placebo-controlled multiple sclerosis clinical trial. Neurology 1994;44(1):16-20.

266.   Poolman R, Struijs P, Krips R, Siervelt I, Marti R, Farrokhyar F, et al. Reporting of outcomes in orthopaedic randomized trials: does blinding of outcome assessors matter? The Journal of Bone and Joint Surgery, American Volume 2007;89(3):550-8.

267.   ICMJE [homepage on the Internet]. ICMJE; 2007 [updated Feb 2006; cited 4 Sept 2007]. [57 screens]. Available from: http://www.icmje.org

268.   Wikipedia, the free encyclopedia [homepage on the Internet]. 2007 [updated 25 Nov 2007; cited 30 Nov 2007]. Effect size; [6 screens]. Available from: http://en.wikipedia.org/wiki/Effect_size

269.   Briand L, El Emam K, Morasca S. On the application of measurement theory in software engineering. Empirical Software Engineering 1995;1(1):61-88.

270.   Levine D. DEA 455/656 research methods in human-environment relations [homepage on the Internet]. Ithaca, USA: Cornell University; [updated unknown; cited 19 Apr 2007]. Measurement scales and statistical analysis; [7 screens]. Available from: http://courses.cit.cornell.edu/dea455/dea455/ho10.pdf

271.   Chuang J, Hripcsak G, Jenders R. Considering clustering: a methodological review of clinical decision support system studies. In: Overhage J, editor. Proceedings of the AMIA 2000 Annual Symposium; Los Angeles, USA. Hanley & Belfus; 2000. p. 146-50.

272.   Dallal G. The little handbook of statistical practice [homepage on the Internet]. Boston, USA: Tufts University; 2007 [updated 11 Aug 2007; cited 21 May 2007]. Units of analysis; [2 screens]. Available from: http://www.tufts.edu/~gdallal/units.htm

273.   Higgins J, Green S, editors. Study designs and identifying the unit of analysis. Cochrane handbook for systematic reviews of interventions 4.2.5 [updated May 2005]; Section 8.3. In The Cochrane Library, Issue 3, 2005. Chichester, UK: John Wiley & Sons, Ltd

274.   Liang K, Zeger S. Longitudinal data analysis using generalized linear models. Biometrika 1986;73(1):13-22.

275.   Horton R, Greenhalgh T. The rhetoric of research - comment/reply. BMJ 1995;310(6985):985.

276.   Kitchenham B. Evaluating software engineering methods and tool part 1: the evaluation context and evaluation methods. Software Engineering Notes 1996;21(1):11-15.

277.   Jarvenpaa S. The importance of laboratory experimentation in IS research (technical correspondence). Communications of the ACM 1988;31(12):1502-4.

278.   Wyatt J, Spiegehalter D. Field trials of medical decision-aids: potential problems and solutions. In: Clayton P, editor. 15th Annual Symposium on Computer Applications in Medical Care; Washington, DC. McGraw-Hill, Inc; 1991. p. 3-7.

279.   Kawamoto K, Houlihan C, Balas A, Lobach D. Improving clinical practice using clinical decision support systems: a systematic review of trials to identify features critical to success. BMJ 2005;330:765.

280.   DSS Research: A Full Service Health Care Marketing Research and Consulting Firm [homepage on the Internet]. Fort Worth, USA: 2006 [updated unknown; cited 30 Jan 2008]. Researcher's Toolkit; [1 screens]. Available from: http://www.dssresearch.com/toolkit/sscalc/size_p2.asp

281.   Bosworth H, Olsen M, Dudley T, Orr M, Neary A, Harrelson M, et al. The Take Control of Your Blood pressure (TCYB) study: study design and methodology. Contemporary Clinical Trials 2007;28(1):33-47.

282.   Bosworth H, Olsen M, McCant F, Harrelson M, Gentry P, Rose C, et al. Hypertension Intervention Nurse Telemedicine Study (HINTS): testing a multifactorial tailored behavioral/educational and a medication management intervention for blood pressure control. The American Heart Journal 2007;153(6):918-24.

283.   Holbrook A, Labiris R, Goldsmith C, Ota K, Harb S, Sebaldt R. Influence of decision aids on patient preferences for anticoagulant therapy: a randomized trial. Canadian Medical Association Journal 2007;176(11):1583-7.

284.   Krist A, Woolf S, Johnson R, Kerns J. Patient education on prostate cancer screening and involvement in decision making. Annals of Family Medicine 2007;5(2):112-9.

285.   Saver B, Gustafson D, Taylor T, Hawkins R, Woods N, Dinauer S, et al. A tale of two studies: the importance of setting, subjects and context in two randomized, controlled trials of a web-based decision support for perimenopausal and postmenopausal health decisions. Patient Education and Counselling 2007;66(2):211-22.

286.   Shulman R, Finney S, O'Sullivan C, Glynne P, Greene R. Tight glycaemic control: a prospective observational study of a computerised decision-supported intensive insulin therapy protocol. Critical Care 2007;11(4):R75.

287.   van Steenkiste B, van der Weijden T, Stoffers H, Kester A, Timmermans D, Grol R. Improving cardiovascular risk management: a randomized, controlled trial on the effect of a decision support tool for patients and physicians. European Journal of Cardiovascular Prevention and Rehabilitation 2007;14(1):44-50.

288.   Zwarenstein M, Dainty K, Quan S, Kiss A, Adhikari N. A cluster randomized trial evaluating electronic prescribing in an ambulatory care setting. Trials 2007;8:28.

289.   Momtahan K, Burns C, Sherrard H, Mesana T, Labinaz M. Using personal digital assistants and patient care algorithms to improve access to cardiac care best practices. Medinfo 2007;12(1):117-21.

290.   Rothschild J, McGurk S, Honour M, Lu L, McClendon A, Srivastava P, et al. Assessment of education and computerized decision support interventions for improving transfusion practice. Transfusion 2007;47(2):228-39.

291.   Albisser A, Wright C, Sakkal S. Averting iatrogenic hypoglycemia through glucose prediction in clinical practice: progress towards a new procedure in diabetes. Diabetes Research and Clinical Practice 2007;76(2):207-14.

292.   Augstein P, Vogt L, Kohnert K, Freyse E, Heinke P, Salzsieder E. Outpatient assessment of Karlsburg Diabetes Management System-based decision support. Diabetes Care 2007;30(7):1704-8.

293.   Col N, Ngo L, Fortin J, Goldberg R, O'Connor A. Can computerized decision support help patients make complex treatment decisions? A randomized controlled trial of an individualized menopause decision aid. Medical Decision Making 2007;27(5):585-98.

294.   Davis R, Wright J, Chalmers F, Levenson L, Brown J, Lozano P, et al. A cluster randomized clinical trial to improve prescribing patterns in ambulatory pediatrics. PLoS Clinical Trials 2007;2(5):e25.

295.   Davison B, Goldenberg S, Wiens K, Gleave M. Comparing a generic and individualized information decision support intervention for men newly diagnosed with localized prostate cancer. Cancer Nursing 2007;30(5):E7-15.

296.   Emery J, Morris H, Goodchild R, Fanshawe T, Prevost A, Bobrow M, et al. The GRAIDS Trial: a cluster randomised controlled trial of computer decision support for the management of familial cancer risk in primary care. British Journal of Cancer 2007;97(4):486-93.

297.   Glassman P, Belperio P, Lanto A, Simon B, Valuck R, Sayers J, et al. The utility of adding retrospective medication profiling to computerized provider order entry in an ambulatory care population. Journal of the American Medical Informatics Association 2007;14(4):424-31.

298.   Kaner E, Heaven B, Rapley T, Murtagh M, Graham R, Thomson R, et al. Medical communication and technology: a video-based process study of the use of decision aids in primary care consultations. BMC Medical Informatics and Decision Making 2007;7(2).

299.   Leibovici L, Paul M, Nielson A, Tacconelli E, Andreassen S. The TREAT project: decision support and prediction using causal probabilistic networks. International Journal of Antimicrobial Agents 2007;20(Suppl 1):S93-102.

300.   Martens J, van der Weijden T, Severens J, de Clercq P, de Bruijn D, Kester A, et al. The effect of computer reminders on GPs' prescribing behaviour: a cluster-randomised trial. International Journal of Medical Informatics 2007;76(3):S403-16.

301.   Montgomery A, Emmett C, Fahey T, Jones C, Ricketts I, Patel R, et al. Two decision aids for mode of delivery among women with previous caesarean section: randomised controlled trial. BMJ 2007;334(7607):1305.

302.   Ozanne E, Annis C, Adduci K, Showstack J, Esserman L. Pilot trial of a computerized decision aid for breast cancer prevention. The Breast Journal 2007;13(2):147-54.

303.   Peterson J, Rosenbaum B, Waitman L, Habermann R, Powers J, Harrell D, et al. Physicians' response to guided geriatric dosing: initial results from a randomized trial. Medinfo 2007;12(2):1037-40.

304.   Protheroe J, Bower P, Chew-Graham C, Peters T, Fahey T. Effectiveness of a computerized decision aid in primary care on decision making and quality of life in menorrhagia: Results of the MENTIP randomized controlled trial. Medical Decision Making 2007;27(5):575-84.

305.   Raebel M, Carrol N, Kelleher J, Chester E, Berga S, Magid D. Randomized trial to improve prescribing safety during pregnancy. Journal of the American Medical Informatics Association 2007;14(4):440-50.

306.   Reeve J, Tenni P, Peterson G. An electronic prompt in dispensing software to promote clinical interventions by community pharmacists: a randomized controlled trial. British Journal of Clinical Pharmacology 2007;DOI:10.1111/j.1365-2125.2007.03012.x.

307.   Schapira M, Gilligan M, McAuliffe T, Garmon G, Carnes M, Nattinger A. Decision-making at menopause: a randomized controlled trial of a computer-based hormone therapy decision-aid. Patient Education and Counselling 2007;67(1-2):100-7.

308.   Taylor B, Dinh M, Kwok R, Dinh D, Chu M, Tan E. Electronic interface for emergency department management of asthma: A randomized control trial of clinician performance. Emergency Medicine Australasia 2007;doi: 10.1111/j.1742-6723.2007.01040.x.

309.   Thomson R, Eccles M, Steen I, Greenaway J, Stobbart L, Murtagh M, et al. A patient decision aid to support shared decision-making on anti-thrombotic treatment of patients with atrial fibrillation: randomised controlled trial. Quality and Safety in Health Care 2007;16(3):216-23.

310.   O'Connor A. Validation of a decisional conflict scale. Medical Decision Making 1995;15(1):25-30.

311.   MeSH [homepage on the Internet]. Bethesda, USA: National Library of Medicine; 1998 [updated unknown; cited 20 Dec 2007]. MeSH; [2 screens]. Available from: http://www.ncbi.nlm.nih.gov/sites/entrez

312.   Liu J, Wyatt J, Altman D. Decision tools in health care: focus on the problem, not the solution. BMC Medical Informatics and Decision Making 2006;6(4).

313.   Lewis D. Evolution of consumer health informatics. CIN 2007;25(6):316.

314.   Akesson K, Saveman B, Nilsson G. Health care consumers' experiences of information communication technology - a summary of literature. International Journal of Medical Informatics 2007;76(9):633-45.

315.   Wikipedia, the free encyclopedia [homepage on the Internet]. 2008 [updated 15 Jul 2008; cited 15 Jul 2008]. Galileo Galilei; [26 screens]. Available from: http://en.wikipedia.org/wiki/Galileo

316.   Wikipedia, the free encyclopedia [homepage on the Internet]. 2008 [updated 17 Jul 2008; cited 19 Jul 2008]. Empirical; [2 screens]. Available from: http://en.wikipedia.org/wiki/Empirical

317.   Wikipedia, the free encyclopedia [homepage on the Internet]. 2008 [updated 16 Jul 2008; cited 19 Jul 2008]. Prothrombin Time; [5 screens]. Available from: http://en.wikipedia.org/wiki/International_normalized_ratio

318.   Wikipedia, the free encyclopedia [homepage on the Internet]. 2008 [updated 28 Jun 2008; cited 19 Jul 2008]. Interactionism; [4 screens]. Available from: http://en.wikipedia.org/wiki/Interactionism

319.   Wikipedia, the free encyclopedia [homepage on the Internet]. 2008 [updated 14 Jul 2008; cited 19 Jul 2008]. Postivism; [9 screens]. Available from: http://en.wikipedia.org/wiki/Postivism

Glossary

Allocation concealment: the process of hiding the knowledge of upcoming experimental group assignment so that investigators cannot subvert the allocation method.

Analysis of variance: a group of statistical methods used to calculate whether several means are different.

Attribute: see construct.

Balancing: the process of assigning equal or near-equal numbers of participants to experimental groups.

Bias: a systematic error.

Blinding: the process of making participants, external assessors or data analysts unaware of experimental group assignment.

Blocking: the process of allocating participants to groups such that the groups are fairly uniform with respect to a certain variable (167). Blocking is synonymous with stratification in this meaning but can also mean the process of balancing (108) (see balancing.)

Boredom effect: a bias of where participants are negatively affected due to maturation (e.g. tedium, length) of the experiment (153) (p. 68).

Carryover effect: a bias where the effect of a treatment in crossover or within-subject experiments persists into the next stage.

Case control study: a type of epidemiological investigation that searches for the relationship between cause and disease by gathering patients with and without the disease and examining whether a cause was present in their pasts.

Categorical measurement: measurement that places objects into categories.

Checklist effect: a bias where participant performance improves due to improved data collection and structure rather than the effect of computerisation (138) (p. 212).

Classical test theory: a group of measurement theories with origins in psychological measurement. A key aspect of classical test theory is that observations contain an error component and a true component.

168

Clinical decision support system: a computer-based tool that processes patient-specific data in order to aid decision making about a patient.

Clinical information system: a computer-based system for managing patient-related data.

Clinical trial: a form of controlled experiment in medicine where patients are allocated to a new medical treatment or the current standard/placebo to examine the benefit of the treatment.

Cohen's kappa: a measure of the chance-corrected agreement between 2 raters for categorical/nominal data (unweighted kappa) or ordinal or discrete interval data (weighted).

Cohort study: a type of epidemiological investigation that searches for the relationship between cause and disease by gathering patients that have and do not have a suspected causative agent for the disease and following them through time to see if the disease develops.

Compensatory equalisation of treatment: a bias where control groups are compensated for not receiving the intervention, and this affects their performance (153) (p. 70).

Compensatory rivalry: a bias where participants not receiving the new treatment are further motivated to demonstrate the current standard is as good (153) (p. 70).

Compliance: the degree to which participants in an experiment adhere to the treatments assigned to them, e.g. taking medicines as instructed in clinical trials or using an information system/software development method as instructed in informatics experiments.

Computer-supported cooperative work: the use of computers for collaboration between individual workers.

Confounding: when the effects of variables on an outcome cannot be distinguished from each other (245) (p. 176).

Construct: the underlying phenomenon or property that a scale/item attempts to measure. This is sometimes also called the latent variable or an attribute.

Contamination: a bias where control and treatment groups become mixed and effectively reduce the size of effect.

Continuous measurement: measurement along a spectrum of an object.

Control group: the experimental group that is the comparison for the group or groups receiving the novel treatment. Control groups usually receive the standard or current level of treatment.

Controlled experiment: a research method to understand cause and effect where objects are manipulated to differ in one aspect (the independent variable) and then compared to each other for the effect on other aspects (dependent variables).

Convenience sampling: sampling of participants into an experiment based on ease of access, e.g. university students. Bias can occur if participants are systematically different to the larger population.

Cronbach's alpha: a measure of the consistency of items within a scale for measuring the same construct (internal consistency).

Crossover study: an experimental design where participants receive all levels of treatment in different stages and act as their own controls. This is a type of within-subject study.

Data completeness effect: an experimental bias where data automatically collected by a computer-based intervention is more complete than that which would have been collected manually (138) (p. 213).

Demonstration study: a study to establish the relationship between variables (138) (p. 365).

Dependent variable: variables in an experiment that are the outcomes measured in response to different treatments. The term is also called a response variable.

Effect size: the size of the relationship between treatments and outcomes.

Empirical: relating to empiricism (truths must be demonstrated by observable evidence.) (316) Experiments are a form of empiricism.

Evaluation: the application of formal methods to understand the merits of an object, usually for the purpose of making decisions about the object.

Exclusion criteria: the criteria by which a participant is denied entry into an experiment.

Expectation effect: a bias when participants' preconceived criticism or enthusiasm for the informatics object or method affects their outcomes.

Experience effect: a bias where a participant experienced with an existing software development method will perform better with than a novel method due to familiarity (152) (p. 117).

Experimental unit: the unit to which a treatment is assigned. In informatics experiments, this is usually an individual person or a small group, e.g. a medical ward team but may also be large organisations. This hierarchy is the level of the unit.

External validity: the extent to which the results of an empirical study are generalisable outside of the study's environment, e.g. across people, place and time.

Fatigue effect: a bias where participants become tired at the later stages of an experiment leading to poorer performance.

Feedback effect: a bias where performance feedback given to participants can improve task performance rather than the effect of a treatment (138) (p. 213).

Generalisability theory: an extension of classical test theories to incorporate different forms of error in measurement.

Hawthorne effect: a bias where the performance of participants in an experiment is increased due to the presence of the investigation rather than the treatment.

History effect: a potential bias when an experiment is carried out at over different points in time (153) (p. 68).

Hypothesis (experimental): a formal statement about the relationship between variables. The null hypothesis states there is no relationship. The alternative hypothesis is the contrary in support of the relationship.

Inclusion criteria: the criteria by which a participant is permitted entry into an experiment.

Independent variable: variables in an experiment that are manipulated for the effect on outcomes. The term is also called a factor or a predictor variable and is often synonymous with treatment.

Index: a measurement instrument for quantifying constructs based on the construct determining or "causing" the indicator. Index can also refer to the actual indicator, e.g. Consumer Price Index. Sometimes the term is used interchangeably with scale (see scale.)

Informatics: the discipline concerned with human and machine processing of information. It includes knowledge from a variety of other fields, e.g. computer science, information science and cognitive science.

Integrated Development Environment: a computer programme that provides various useful software development functions, e.g. graphical interface, editor, compiler and debugger.

Intention to treat analysis: a statistical approach in clinical trials where all patients are analysed according to their original group assignments whether or not compliance with treatment occurred.

Internal replication: replication of an experiment by the same researchers.

Internal validity: the extent to which the results of an empirical study are truthful.

International Normalized Ratio: a standardised measure of the clotting ability of blood (317).

Interpretivism: the philosophical view that knowledge is interpreted by observers and is achieved by social interaction (318).

Intraclass correlation coefficient: a group of measures that examines the relationship among multiple observations of the same variable (131) (p. 133).

Item: the part of a scale that seeks a response from the scale user. An item is often comprised of a question (the stem) and a way for users to respond (the response). For continuous responses, each unit of response is called a response step.

Journal Impact Factor: for a given journal and year, the ratio of the number of citations in that year to articles published in the journal during the previous 2 years over the number of citable sources published in the same 2 years (251).

Known-groups validity: a method of validity testing where an instrument is applied to previously categorised groups to see whether it can similarly discriminate.

Lab package: the collection of documentation and experimental materials used in software engineering experiments for other researchers to conduct similar studies.

Learning effect: a bias where participants learn an experimental task, computing artefact or method; performance may improve from learning rather than the experimental treatment. Alternatively, performance may be hindered by insufficient learning of tasks or objects.

Measurement study: a study undertaken to assess the error associated with a measurement instrument (138) (p. 369).

Mono-method bias: bias resulting from the use of a single type of observation whose measurement may be erroneous (153) (p. 71).

Mono-operation bias: bias resulting from an overly simplified experiment that is not representative of what the experiment is trying to show (153) (p. 71).

Monotonic function: a mathematical function that transforms a set of values in a purely increasing or decreasing manner such that ranking is preserved.

Negative finding (result): an experimental result where the intervention was inferior to the control. Sometimes this term is confusingly used to mean a null result, i.e. statistically nonsignificant; therefore, efficacy remains unknown.

Novelty effect: a bias where participants' behaviour changes due to the novelty of the treatment or experimental environment rather than the treatment itself.

Number needed to treat: a measure in clinical trials of the effectiveness of therapies. It is the number of patients who need to be treated to prevent a single adverse health outcome.

Observer bias: a bias where external assessors of an outcome are influenced in their estimation by knowledge of group assignment.

Parallel-group study: an experimental design where single treatment levels are assigned to individual groups that are studied in parallel.

Participant: a human subject enrolled into an experiment.

Placebo effect: a bias where participant outcomes are overestimated due to the positive expectations surrounding a novel intervention, e.g. a new drug or information technology (see expectation effect.)

Positivism: the philosophical view that knowledge is scientific, measurable, objective, reducible and testable (319).

Pseudorandom (allocation): methods of allocating participants to experimental groups based on things that appear random but are partly systematic.

Psychometrics: the discipline concerned with measurement of social and psychological phenomena.

Qualitative: relating to subjective assessment.

Quantitative: relating to quantifiable assessment.

Randomisation: the process of allocating participants to experiment groups according to chance.

Recall error: a bias where participants are required to remember an outcome that may be systematically easier to recall depending on the outcome or its association with other factors, e.g. critical clinicians using a CDSS may remember adverse health outcomes associated with its use more than control clinicians recalling their outcomes.

Reliability coefficient: a numerical value of the consistency of a measurement.

Reliability: the property of a measurement to be consistent or free of error.

Resentful demoralisation: an opposite bias to compensatory rivalry where participants not receiving the novel treatment become unmotivated and perform poorly (153) (p .70).

Sampling (experimental): the process by which participants may be selected to enter an experiment from a larger population.

Scale: an instrument consisting of one or more items, which are scored, and is used to measure the degree of variables "not readily observable by direct means." (125) (p. 8) Scale is sometimes used to distinctly mean a unidimensional instrument (see index.) Scale can also be synonymous with level of measurement or refer to the format of item responses, e.g. "measured on a bipolar scale."

Scientific method: an approach to knowledge discovery by observation, formulation of hypotheses and testing of hypotheses by empirical and, usually, experimental methods.

Second-look bias: a bias where participants are asked to review a case scenario without the use of an informational tool and then with tool. Outcomes may improve from the second chance to think about the case rather than the tool's use (138) (p. 215).

Selection effect (bias): a bias where factors relating to the entry of participants affect the outcomes of an experiment rather than the treatment, e.g. volunteers are usually more motivated, which could affect performance (153) (p. 69). Bias can also reflect poor representativeness of the sample. Bias can also occur from nonrandom allocation to experimental groups, i.e. biased selection into groups.

Setting effect: a bias where the experimental setting, e.g. time of day, can adversely affect participant performance.

Statistical regression effect: a bias when participants are allocated treatment based on classification by a previous study. A change in outcomes can occur due to the classification scheme rather than the treatment (153) (p. 69).

Stratification: see blocking.

Task: see test case.

Test case: the scenarios against which human/machine information processing or skill is applied. These can also include tasks.

Test-retest method: a form of reliability testing where objects are assessed at different points in time; measurements on the same object are compared for consistency.

Treatment level: the possible values of a treatment (or independent variable), e.g. if the independent variable is provision of informational support, one treatment may be a computer programme, another may be a paper guideline and another treatment level may be nothing (control).

Treatment: the aspect of experimental groups that is manipulated to see its relationship to outcomes of interest. This is often synonymous with independent variable. However, treatments can also be the possible values that an independent variable can take in an experiment (152) (p. 60). A "treatment group" is often distinguished from a "control group" by the level of the treatment (see treatment level and independent variable).

Triangulation: the use of different investigations or methods to check for consistency of an object of study (138) (p. 262).

Type I error: the mistaken rejection of the null hypothesis when it is, in fact, true.

Type II error: the mistaken acceptance of the null hypothesis when it is, in fact, false.

Unconscious formalisation: a bias in within-subject studies where formalised software development methods are learned from one part of an experiment and structure the control situation (use of less formal techniques) (152) (p. 118).

Unit of analysis error: a statistical error when analysis does not take into account clustering of data and loss of independence and, therefore, inflates sample sizes. As a result, confidence intervals become artificially narrowed and tests of inference may become erroneously significant.

Unit of analysis: the unit in an experiment that is the object of statistical methods. To prevent unit of analysis error, it should be the same as the experimental unit.

Unit of observation: the unit in an experiment that an observation is made upon. To prevent unit of analysis error, it should be the same as the experimental unit.

Validity: the property of a measurement to truly capture that which it is supposed to measure.

Withdrawal: a participant who is assigned to an experimental group but does not complete the experiment. This is also called a dropout.

Within-subject study: an experimental design where participants act as their own controls (see crossover study.)

Appendices

Appendix A contains the spreadsheet data of pooled experimental concepts and endorsing sources. # indicates stated endorsement of a concept or semantic equivalent. ~ indicates indirect endorsement (not directly stated but implied in other statements). The textbook by Juristo and Moreno describes important experimental concepts in a chapter on recommendations/guidelines (p. 349-58) and in the rest of the text. * indicates endorsement in other chapters of that textbook (152).

Appendix B lists the MICE-80 questionnaire items that were dropped to produce the MICE-38 version.

Appendix C contains the raw data produced from testing validity of the MICE-80 and MICE-38 questionnaire versions.

Appendix D displays the raw item responses for the review of clinical decision support tool experiments in Chapter 5.

INTRODUCTION	What is the problem the study addresses, its motivation	What is the object of study, e.g. product, process, model	What is the level of industrial use of the object of study	Aim for replicated studies	Is the study compared to current knowledge, underlying theory	Is the underlying theory insufficiently defined	Is it a non-trivial study	Was there a description of the tasks the technology or process addresses	Is experiment or study design most appropriate	Is the study appropriate for system maturity
COMPUTER SCIENCE Basili 1986 (158)	#	#		#	#					
Basili 1999 (159)	#	#		#	#					
Boudreau (160)										
Brooks (161)										
Fenton (16)										
Host (162)										
Jarvenpaa (163)				~	#		#			
Jedlitschka (113)	#	#			#					
Juristo 2001 (152)	#	#*		#	#		#			
Juristo 2004 (164)				#	~				~	
Kitchenham 2002 (122)					#		#			
Kitchenham 2006 (165)			#		#			#		
Lott (166)	#	#		#	#				#	
Moher 1981 (100)										
Moher 1982 (80)										

Pfleeger (167-170)		#		#				#	
Sadler (123)									
Singer (114)	#				#				
Sjoberg (94)									
Weinberg (119)					#	~			
Wohlin (153)	#	#		#	#	#		#	
HEALTH INFORMATICS Balas (146)									
Johnston (171)									
Friedman (138)	#				#		#	#	#
MEDICINE Altman (108)	#				#				
Chalmers 1990 (172)									
Chalmers 1981 (142)									
Cho (173)	#							#	
Colditz (174)									
Detsky (175)									
Evans (176)									
Goodman (143)	#				#		~		
Imperiale (177)									
Jadad (141)									
Kleijnen (178)									
Reisch (179)	#								
Verhagen (180)									

METHOD	Is there a definition of aims, objectives or goals	Is there a formal hypotheses	Are the methods reproducible	What is the perspective of the study	Has a pilot study been done	Aim for within-subject designs	Was there a prospective study of hazards
COMPUTER SCIENCE Basili 1986 (158)	#			#	#		
Basili 1999 (159)	#	#	~	#			
Boudreau (160)					#		
Brooks (161)						#	
Fenton (16)							
Host (162)							
Jarvenpaa (163)					#		
Jedlitschka (113)	#	#	~	#			
Juristo 2001 (152)	#	#					
Juristo 2004 (164)			~				
Kitchenham 2002 (122)	#	#					
Kitchenham 2006 (165)							
Lott (166)	#	#		#			
Moher 1981 (100)					#		
Moher 1982 (80)							
Pfleeger (167-170)	#	#			#		
Sadler (123)							

Singer (114)	#	#	~				
Sjoberg (94)							
Weinberg (119)							
Wohlin (153)	#	#	#	#			
HEALTH INFORMATICS Balas (146)							
Johnston (171)							
Friedman (138)	#		#	#	#		
MEDICINE Altman (108)	#	#					
Chalmers 1990 (172)							
Chalmers 1981 (142)							
Cho (173)	#						
Colditz (174)							
Detsky (175)							
Evans (176)		#					
Goodman (143)	#	#					
Imperiale (177)							
Jadad (141)							
Kleijnen (178)							
Reisch (179)	#						#
Verhagen (180)							

STUDY DESIGN	Is the design correct for the hypothesis	Aim for simple study design	Avoid simple designs, e.g. one factor	Use more than 1 independent variable	Was there a description of who did the monitoring	Was there a description of study design	Has balancing been described	Were carryover or refractory effects considered	Was there a description of internal replication	Was scheduling reported	Was the study long enough	Evaluate against current practice
COMPUTER SCIENCE Basili 1986 (158)						#						
Basili 1999 (159)						~		#				#
Boudreau (160)												
Brooks (161)												
Fenton (16)	#										#	
Host (162)	#										#	
Jarvenpaa (163)			#	#								
Jedlitschka (113)		#				#	#			#		
Juristo 2001 (152)	#*		#*	#*	#	#*			#	#		
Juristo 2004 (164)	~											
Kitchenham 2002 (122)	#	#				#		#				#
Kitchenham 2006 (165)												
Lott (166)					~	#				#		
Moher 1981 (100)												
Moher 1982 (80)												
Pfleeger (167-170)	#	#				#	#					
Sadler (123)												

	1	2	3	4	5	6	7	8	9	10	11	12	13
Singer (114)							#	#					
Sjoberg (94)												#	
Weinberg (119)													
Wohlin (153)	#	#	#	#			#	#					
HEALTH INFORMATICS Balas (146)											#		
Johnston (171)													
Friedman (138)	~						#		#		#		
MEDICINE Altman (108)						#	~	~			#		
Chalmers 1990 (172)													
Chalmers 1981 (142)						#	#				#		
Cho (173)							#						
Colditz (174)													
Detsky (175)													
Evans (176)													
Goodman (143)	~						#				#		
Imperiale (177)													
Jadad (141)													
Kleijnen (178)													
Reisch (179)						~			#				
Verhagen (180)													

BLOCKING	Were the control and treatment groups comparable	Were comparable materials or co-interventions used except where experimentally manipulated	Was there control or analysis for multiple measured variables, e.g. stratify, regression	Were known confounders handled in design or analysis	Were known risk factors recorded	Was there a description of unchanging characteristics (parameters)	Was there a description of blocking variables (stratification)	Was the sample uniform
COMPUTER SCIENCE Basili 1986 (158)								
Basili 1999 (159)								
Boudreau (160)								
Brooks (161)		#					#	#
Fenton (16)								
Host (162)								
Jarvenpaa (163)	~	#	~	#	~			
Jedlitschka (113)							#	
Juristo 2001 (152)	#		~*	~*		#	#	~*
Juristo 2004 (164)								
Kitchenham 2002 (122)	#							
Kitchenham 2006 (165)								
Lott (166)	~			~			#	
Moher 1981 (100)								#
Moher 1982 (80)								
Pfleeger (167-170)				#			#	
Sadler (123)								

Singer (114)								
Sjoberg (94)								
Weinberg (119)								
Wohlin (153)	~						#	#
HEALTH INFORMATICS Balas (146)	#							
Johnston (171)	#			#				
Friedman (138)								
MEDICINE Altman (108)	#	#					#	
Chalmers 1990 (172)	#							
Chalmers 1981 (142)	#	~						
Cho (173)	~			#				
Colditz (174)								
Detsky (175)								
Evans (176)	#	#	#		#			#
Goodman (143)	#	~	#	~	~			
Imperiale (177)	#	#						
Jadad (141)								
Kleijnen (178)								
Reisch (179)	#	#		#			~	#
Verhagen (180)	#			~	~			

BIASES	Was there control of checklist effect	Was there control of data completeness effect	Was there control of feedback effect	Was there control of placebo effect	Describe the placebo characteristics. Was it identical to treatment	Was there control of second-look bias	Was there control of testing-treatment interactions	Was there control of interaction of different treatments	Was there control of experience effect	Was conformance or compliance assessed	Was there control of unconscious formalisation effect	Was there control of setting effect	Was there control of novelty effect	Were random irrelevancies accounted for
COMPUTER SCIENCE Basili 1986 (158)														
Basili 1999 (159)										#				
Boudreau (160)														
Brooks (161)														
Fenton (16)														
Host (162)														
Jarvenpaa (163)														
Jedlitschka (113)										#				
Juristo 2001 (152)			#*						#*	#*	#	#	#	
Juristo 2004 (164)														
Kitchenham 2002 (122)										~				
Kitchenham 2006 (165)														
Lott (166)										#				

Moher 1981 (100)														
Moher 1982 (80)														
Pfleeger (167-170)														
Sadler (123)				#									#	
Singer (114)														
Sjoberg (94)														
Weinberg (119)														
Wohlin (153)						#	#		#					#
HEALTH INFORMATICS Balas (146)							~							
Johnston (171)														
Friedman (138)	#	#	#	#		#								
MEDICINE Altman (108)				#	#									
Chalmers 1990 (172)				#	#									
Chalmers 1981 (142)				#	#				#					
Cho (173)				#										
Colditz (174)				#										
Detsky (175)														
Evans (176)														
Goodman (143)				#					~					
Imperiale (177)														
Jadad (141)				#	#									
Kleijnen (178)				#	#									
Reisch (179)				#	#				#					
Verhagen (180)				#										

BIASES (CONTINUED)	Was there control of selection effect, e.g. volunteers	Was there control of Hawthorne effect	Was there control of learning effect	Was there control of boredom effect	Was there control of statistical regression effect	Prevent intergroup communication (including contamination)	Was there control of compensatory equalization of treatments	Was there control of compensatory rivalry	Was there control of resentful demoralization	Was there control of history effects	Were subjects biased for or against the treatment	Was measurement bias accounted for by methods other than blinding	Are the investigators studying their own work	Avoid mono-operation bias	Avoid use of a single type of measure (mono-method bias)	Does the investigator teach technology of study to student subjects
COMPUTER SCIENCE Basili 1986 (158)																
Basili 1999 (159)			#	#												
Boudreau (160)																
Brooks (161)																
Fenton (16)																
Host (162)											~					
Jarvenpaa (163)			#													
Jedlitschka (113)																
Juristo 2001 (152)			#	#	#*						~					
Juristo 2004 (164)																
Kitchenham 2002 (122)			#									#	#			
Kitchenham 2006 (165)																
Lott (166)			#									#				

	1	2	3	4	5	6	7	8	9	10	11	12	13	14	15
Moher 1981 (100)															
Moher 1982 (80)			#								~				
Pfleeger (167-170)															
Sadler (123)		#	#								#			~	~
Singer (114)															
Sjoberg (94)						#									#
Weinberg (119)		#	#												
Wohlin (153)	#	#	#	#	#	#	#	#	#	#	#		#	#	#
HEALTH INFORMATICS Balas (146)															
Johnston (171)												~			
Friedman (138)	#	#				#					~		#		
MEDICINE Altman (108)															
Chalmers 1990 (172)															
Chalmers 1981 (142)							#								
Cho (173)												#			
Colditz (174)															
Detsky (175)															
Evans (176)															
Goodman (143)															
Imperiale (177)												~			
Jadad (141)															
Kleijnen (178)															
Reisch (179)															
Verhagen (180)															

TREATMETN AND SETTING	Was there a description of treatment	Were the treatment levels defined	Is the treatment appropriate for questions posed	Was there an attempt to measure the available therapeutic agent	Was there a description of the site	Was the setting representative
COMPUTER SCIENCE Basili 1986 (158)						
Basili 1999 (159)	#				#	#
Boudreau (160)						
Brooks (161)			#			
Fenton (16)						~
Host (162)						
Jarvenpaa (163)						
Jedlitschka (113)	#	#			#	
Juristo 2001 (152)	#	#	#			
Juristo 2004 (164)						#
Kitchenham 2002 (122)	#				#	
Kitchenham 2006 (165)	#	#				
Lott (166)	#				#	
Moher 1981 (100)						

Moher 1982 (80)	#	#			#	#
Pfleeger (167-170)	#					
Sadler (123)						
Singer (114)	#					
Sjoberg (94)						#
Weinberg (119)						
Wohlin (153)	#	#	#		#	#
HEALTH INFORMATICS Balas (146)	#				#	
Johnston (171)						
Friedman (138)	#	~			#	
MEDICINE Altman (108)	#				#	
Chalmers 1990 (172)						
Chalmers 1981 (142)	#	#		#	#	
Cho (173)						
Colditz (174)						
Detsky (175)	#	~				
Evans (176)	#	~	#			
Goodman (143)					#	
Imperiale (177)			#			
Jadad (141)						
Kleijnen (178)	#	~				
Reisch (179)	#	#	#			
Verhagen (180)						

PARTICIPANTS	Was there a description of the sampling method (including eligibility criteria)	Were the subjects suitable for questions posed	Was the student vs. professional issue addressed	Were motivation issues addressed	Are sample characteristics adequately described	Avoid disturbing or interrupting subjects	Was group over individual effects studied	Are the controls appropriate	Were controls adequately defined	Avoid using controls if control situation is ambiguous	Was the experimental unit defined	Select subjects prior to treatment and evaluate prospectively	Was the sample representative	Reassure subjects that their performance is not the main outcome
COMPUTER SCIENCE Basili 1986 (158)													#	
Basili 1999 (159)		~	#	#	#								#	
Boudreau (160)														
Brooks (161)		~	#										#	
Fenton (16)													~	
Host (162)		~	#	#	#									
Jarvenpaa (163)					~			~	~					
Jedlitschka (113)	#	~		#	#									
Juristo 2001 (152)	#	~		#	#	#*			~		#			#*
Juristo 2004 (164)													~	
Kitchenham 2002 (122)	#	~	#		#					#	#		#	
Kitchenham 2006 (165)											#			
Lott (166)	#	~	#	#	#									

192

Moher 1981 (100)		~	#		#							
Moher 1982 (80)	#	~	#	#	#				#			
Pfleeger (167-170)	#				#			#	#			
Sadler (123)		~		#								
Singer (114)	#	~		#	#							
Sjoberg (94)		~	#	#	#							#
Weinberg (119)		~	#				#					
Wohlin (153)		~	~	#	#			~				#
HEALTH INFORMATICS Balas (146)	#											
Johnston (171)									#			
Friedman (138)	#				#			#	#	#		
MEDICINE Altman (108)	#				#			#				
Chalmers 1990 (172)												
Chalmers 1981 (142)	#											
Cho (173)	#						#				#	
Colditz (174)	#											
Detsky (175)	#							#				
Evans (176)	#				#		~	#				
Goodman (143)	#				#			#	#			
Imperiale (177)	#											
Jadad (141)												
Kleijnen (178)					#							
Reisch (179)	#	#			#			~			#	#
Verhagen (180)	#											

RANDOMISATION AND BLINDING	Was there a description of randomisation or allocation of treatment	Has allocation concealment been done	Separate person for allocation generation and implementation	Did the investigators randomise as late as possible	Was randomisation checked	Was analysis blinded	Was blinding checked	Were participants blinded to treatment group	Were the subjects blinded to hypotheses	Were outcome assessors blinded to treatment group	Were health providers blinded to treatment group	Explain why blinding was not used	Use of blind allocation of materials
COMPUTER SCIENCE Basili 1986 (158)													
Basili 1999 (159)													
Boudreau (160)													
Brooks (161)													
Fenton (16)													
Host (162)													
Jarvenpaa (163)													
Jedlitschka (113)	#					#		~		~			
Juristo 2001 (152)	#								#*				
Juristo 2004 (164)													
Kitchenham 2002 (122)	#					#				#			#
Kitchenham 2006 (165)													
Lott (166)	#												
Moher 1981 (100)													

Moher 1982 (80)	#											
Pfleeger (167-170)	#											
Sadler (123)							#		#			
Singer (114)	#											
Sjoberg (94)												
Weinberg (119)												
Wohlin (153)	#								#			
HEALTH INFORMATICS Balas (146)	#	~	~		#			#		#	#	
Johnston (171)	#									#		
Friedman (138)	#	#		#				#		#	#	
MEDICINE Altman (108)	#	#	#			#	#	#		#	#	#
Chalmers 1990 (172)	#	#						#		#	#	
Chalmers 1981 (142)	#	#			#	#	#	#			#	
Cho (173)	#							#		#		
Colditz (174)	#	#						#		#		
Detsky (175)	#	#								#		
Evans (176)	~	#								#		
Goodman (143)	#						#	#		#	#	
Imperiale (177)										~		
Jadad (141)	#	#						#		#		
Kleijnen (178)	#						#	#		~	~	
Reisch (179)	#	#					#	#		#	#	
Verhagen (180)	#	#						#		#	#	

MATERIALS AND TASKS/TEST CASES	Was there a description of examination materials (including training, aids)	Were materials representative	Use measures of computer programme complexity	Appropriate level of task difficulty to achieve statistical normality	Appropriate level of task difficulty to distinguish ability	Tasks familiar or easy enough for subjects to understand	Was there variety and sufficient number of test cases	Were test cases comprehensive	Were test cases recent and geographically distinct	Were task constraints defined	Were tasks clearly defined	Were tasks representative
COMPUTER SCIENCE Basili 1986 (158)												
Basili 1999 (159)	#	~										~
Boudreau (160)												
Brooks (161)		#	#	#								
Fenton (16)		~										~
Host (162)												
Jarvenpaa (163)	#					#					#	
Jedlitschka (113)	#											
Juristo 2001 (152)	#											
Juristo 2004 (164)		#										#
Kitchenham 2002 (122)		#										
Kitchenham 2006 (165)												
Lott (166)	#											
Moher 1981 (100)		#			#							#

Moher 1982 (80)	#	#									#	#	#
Pfleeger (167-170)	#												
Sadler (123)													
Singer (114)	#												
Sjoberg (94)		#											#
Weinberg (119)	~												
Wohlin (153)	#	~											~
HEALTH INFORMATICS Balas (146)													
Johnston (171)													
Friedman (138)								#	#	#			#
MEDICINE Altman (108)													
Chalmers 1990 (172)													
Chalmers 1981 (142)													
Cho (173)													
Colditz (174)													
Detsky (175)													
Evans (176)													
Goodman (143)													
Imperiale (177)													
Jadad (141)													
Kleijnen (178)													
Reisch (179)													
Verhagen (180)													

OUTCOMES	Was there a description of outcomes	Was there a description of instrumentation (guidelines, measurement)	Was data collection planned prior to treatment and collected prospectively	Was there a description of data collection procedures or evaluation methods	Were the measures tested for content, criterion, construct validity	Was a measurement study done prior to demonstration study	Avoid oversimplification of outcomes	Were outcome measures justified	Were correct clinical investigations used	Were outcome measures validated	Are validated measurement tools re-used	Was there a prior estimate of improvement	Was there use of both qualitative and quantitative data	Objective measures preferable to subjective	Were outcomes defined prior to study	Use of outcomes of interest to practitioners
COMPUTER SCIENCE Basili 1986 (158)	#			#						#						
Basili 1999 (159)	#			#						#						
Boudreau (160)		~		#	#	#				#	#					
Brooks (161)																
Fenton (16)								#						#		
Host (162)								#						#		
Jarvenpaa (163)					#	#				#	#					
Jedlitschka (113)	#	#		#				#		#	#					
Juristo 2001 (152)	#	#		#	~ *			#		# *			#*	#		
Juristo 2004 (164)																#
Kitchenham 2002 (122)	#			#		#	#	#		#					~	
Kitchenham 2006 (165)	#															
Lott (166)	#	~		#						#		#				

198

Moher 1981 (100)											#			
Moher 1982 (80)	#							#	#		#		#	
Pfleeger (167-170)	#			#										
Sadler (123)														
Singer (114)	#													
Sjoberg (94)														
Weinberg (119)							#	~						
Wohlin (153)	#	#		#					#				#	
HEALTH INFORMATICS Balas (146)	#										#			
Johnston (171)	#			#									#	
Friedman (138)	#	#		#	#	#			#	#		#		
MEDICINE Altman (108)	#				~				#	#	#			#
Chalmers 1990 (172)														
Chalmers 1981 (142)	~								#		#			
Cho (173)														#
Colditz (174)														
Detsky (175)				#									#	
Evans (176)	#			~				#			#			
Goodman (143)	#							#						
Imperiale (177)													~	
Jadad (141)														
Kleijnen (178)	#			~										#
Reisch (179)	#		#	#	~				#		#		#	
Verhagen (180)														

RESULTS	Were magnitude of effects reported	Describe how the experiment actually executed	Describe how exceptions to study design were handled	Are the results presented	Is baseline clinical or demographic data provided	Is there a participant flow description	Report number needed to treat	Were relevant subgroup effects explored in appropriate detail	Subgroup analyses should be prespecified and justified	Were raw data included	Were descriptive statistics included	Report summary statistics for diagnostic tests (sensitivity etc)	Was the data set validity assessed (e.g. outliers)	Is there a description of timing of outcomes	Avoid unjustified precision	Was there a description of adverse effects	Was there a life-table or time-series analysis	Is there analysis of secondary variables (interactions, side effects)
COMPUTER SCIENCE Basili 1986 (158)		#		#														
Basili 1999 (159)																		
Boudreau (160)																		
Brooks (161)																		
Fenton (16)																		
Host (162)																		
Jarvenpaa (163)																		
Jedlitschka (113)		#	#	#							#	#		#				
Juristo 2001 (152)	~		#	#								#*						
Juristo 2004 (164)																		
Kitchenham 2002 (122)	#		#	~							#	#		#		#	#	
Kitchenham 2006 (165)														#				
Lott (166)			#								#			#				
Moher 1981 (100)																		

200

	1	2	3	4	5	6	7	8	9	10	11	12	13	14	15	16	17	18
Moher 1982 (80)																		
Pfleeger (167-170)			#										#					
Sadler (123)																		
Singer (114)		~		#							#							
Sjoberg (94)																		
Weinberg (119)															#			
Wohlin (153)		#		#							#		#					
HEALTH INFORMATICS Balas (146)	#			#							#					#		#
Johnston (171)					~													
Friedman (138)				#			#									#		
MEDICINE Altman (108)	#	~		~	#	#	#		#		#			#		#		#
Chalmers 1990 (172)																		
Chalmers 1981 (142)				#	#				~					#		#	#	#
Cho (173)																#		
Colditz (174)	#			#														
Detsky (175)																		
Evans (176)				#	#				#							#		
Goodman (143)	#			#	#			#				#				#		
Imperiale (177)																		
Jadad (141)																		
Kleijnen (178)										~	#							
Reisch (179)											#					#		
Verhagen (180)	#			#														

WITHDRAWALS AND INELIGIBILITY	Were all eligible subjects enrolled	Were there specific procedures to minimise loss	Was there a description of not eligible or eligible who refused	Was there a description of withdrawals	Was there a comparison of non-participants to participants	Adequate ratio of retained subjects	Were withdrawals or missing data analysed correctly
COMPUTER SCIENCE Basili 1986 (158)							
Basili 1999 (159)							
Boudreau (160)							
Brooks (161)							
Fenton (16)							
Host (162)							
Jarvenpaa (163)							
Jedlitschka (113)							
Juristo 2001 (152)							#*
Juristo 2004 (164)							
Kitchenham 2002 (122)		#			#		#
Kitchenham 2006 (165)							
Lott (166)							

Moher 1981 (100)								
Moher 1982 (80)								
Pfleeger (167-170)								
Sadler (123)								
Singer (114)								
Sjoberg (94)								
Weinberg (119)								
Wohlin (153)			#					
HEALTH INFORMATICS Balas (146)			#	#		#	#	
Johnston (171)						#		
Friedman (138)								
MEDICINE Altman (108)			~	~				
Chalmers 1990 (172)				#		#	#	
Chalmers 1981 (142)			#	#	#	#	#	
Cho (173)				#				
Colditz (174)	#			#				
Detsky (175)			#					
Evans (176)				#		#		
Goodman (143)			#	#	#		#	
Imperiale (177)								
Jadad (141)				#				
Kleijnen (178)								
Reisch (179)		#	#	#				~
Verhagen (180)								

203

STATISTICAL METHODS	If Bayesian methods used, seek statistician	Was a statistician sought	Was there a sample size assessment	Give reasons for deviations from calculated sample size	Was error estimated by a measurement study included in results	Was level of measurement correct	Higher level of measurement preferable	Was there a description or reference for statistical procedures	Avoid unit of analysis error	Was there ignorance of trend in results (no interim analyses or multiple looks) or prespecified correction	Appropriate retrospective analyses (post-hoc subgroups)	Was there use of hypothesis testing	Remove redundant data	Avoid or adjust for fishing for results, too many tests	Are the statistical methods appropriate
COMPUTER SCIENCE Basili 1986 (158)															#
Basili 1999 (159)															
Boudreau (160)															
Brooks (161)			#												
Fenton (16)						#	#								#
Host (162)						#	#								#
Jarvenpaa (163)															
Jedlitschka (113)		#	#			~		#				#			#
Juristo 2001 (152)			#*			#		#				#*			#
Juristo 2004 (164)															~
Kitchenham 2002 (122)	#	#	#			~		#	#					#	#
Kitchenham 2006 (165)															
Lott (166)			#			~						#		#	#
Moher 1981 (100)			#												

204

	1	2	3	4	5	6	7	8	9	10	11	12	13	14	15
Moher 1982 (80)		#													
Pfleeger (167-170)	#	#										#			#
Sadler (123)															
Singer (114)							#								#
Sjoberg (94)															
Weinberg (119)															
Wohlin (153)		#		#	#	#						#	#	#	#
HEALTH INFORMATICS Balas (146)		#							#	#	#				
Johnston (171)								~							
Friedman (138)	#	#		#	#	#	#	#							#
MEDICINE Altman (108)		#	#				#		#	#				#	~
Chalmers 1990 (172)															
Chalmers 1981 (142)	#	#					#		#	#					#
Cho (173)		#					#								#
Colditz (174)							#								
Detsky (175)		#					#								#
Evans (176)		#					#		#					#	#
Goodman (143)		~			#			#							#
Imperiale (177)															
Jadad (141)															
Kleijnen (178)		~													
Reisch (179)		#					#		#	#				#	#
Verhagen (180)															

STATISTICAL METHODS (CONTINUED)	Statistical analysis beyond means, percentages, standard deviations	Use of regression or correlation as appropriate	Choose significance level before commencing experiment	Are confidence limits included	Were negative results assessed for type II error	Was type I error considered	Was intention to treat analysis used	Were statistical test constraints obeyed	Report statistical package	Apply both parametric and nonparametric tests and compare
COMPUTER SCIENCE Basili 1986 (158)		~						#		
Basili 1999 (159)										
Boudreau (160)										
Brooks (161)										
Fenton (16)										
Host (162)										
Jarvenpaa (163)										
Jedlitschka (113)	~			#				#		
Juristo 2001 (152)					#*	#		#		#
Juristo 2004 (164)										
Kitchenham 2002 (122)				#				#	#	
Kitchenham 2006 (165)										
Lott (166)	~		#		#	#				

Moher 1981 (100)										
Moher 1982 (80)				#						
Pfleeger (167-170)	~	#						#		
Sadler (123)										
Singer (114)										
Sjoberg (94)										
Weinberg (119)										
Wohlin (153)					#	#		#		
HEALTH INFORMATICS Balas (146)	~			#		#				
Johnston (171)										
Friedman (138)					#	#	#	#		
MEDICINE Altman (108)	~			#	#	#	#	#		
Chalmers 1990 (172)						#				
Chalmers 1981 (142)	~	#		#	#	#	#			
Cho (173)				#	#					
Colditz (174)	#								#	
Detsky (175)	~			#	#					
Evans (176)				#	#	#		#		
Goodman (143)				#		#				
Imperiale (177)										
Jadad (141)										
Kleijnen (178)				#						
Reisch (179)				#	#	#	#			
Verhagen (180)				#		#				

DISCUSSION	Did the investigators critically analyse their study	Was there consideration of deterministic vs. probabilistic causality	Was there interpretation of results and do results justify conclusions	Is the study externally valid	Was there consideration of causal direction	Do they distinguish statistical significance vs. practical importance	Was there an assessment of negative findings	Was there an assessment of unexpected findings	Avoid dwelling on unexpected findings	Do the investigators describe further experiments
COMPUTER SCIENCE Basili 1986 (158)			#	~						
Basili 1999 (159)				#						
Boudreau (160)										
Brooks (161)										
Fenton (16)				#						
Host (162)				~						
Jarvenpaa (163)										
Jedlitschka (113)	#		#	#			#	#		#
Juristo 2001 (152)		#*	#	#*						#
Juristo 2004 (164)			#	#						
Kitchenham 2002 (122)	#		#	#		#	#			
Kitchenham 2006 (165)										
Lott (166)			#	#						

	1	2	3	4	5	6	7	8	9	10
Moher 1981 (100)				#						
Moher 1982 (80)										
Pfleeger (167-170)										
Sadler (123)										
Singer (114)			#						#	
Sjoberg (94)				#						
Weinberg (119)				#						
Wohlin (153)	#		#	#	#	#				#
HEALTH INFORMATICS Balas (146)										
Johnston (171)										
Friedman (138)	#		#	#		#				
MEDICINE Altman (108)	#		#	#		#	#			
Chalmers 1990 (172)										
Chalmers 1981 (142)			#				#			
Cho (173)			#	#		~	#			
Colditz (174)			#							
Detsky (175)							#			
Evans (176)			#			~				
Goodman (143)	#		#	#						
Imperiale (177)										
Jadad (141)										
Kleijnen (178)										
Reisch (179)			#	#						
Verhagen (180)										

PRESENTATION	Is the abstract accurate	Are graphics, figures, tables used appropriately	Was there a reporting structure (e.g. abstract, IMRAD, references, appendix)	Was IMRAD used	Is reporting redundant	Is there a balance between detail and summary results	Is the reporting complete	Are there inaccuracies in the report	Are computation errors/contradictions present	Do comparisons use same number of subjects, if not then explained
COMPUTER SCIENCE Basili 1986 (158)										
Basili 1999 (159)										
Boudreau (160)										
Brooks (161)										
Fenton (16)										
Host (162)										
Jarvenpaa (163)										
Jedlitschka (113)	~		#				~			
Juristo 2001 (152)			#							
Juristo 2004 (164)										
Kitchenham 2002 (122)		#								
Kitchenham 2006 (165)					#	#				
Lott (166)										
Moher 1981 (100)										
Moher 1982 (80)										
Pfleeger (167-170)			#							

Sadler (123)											
Singer (114)	#		#	#				~			
Sjoberg (94)											
Weinberg (119)											
Wohlin (153)		#	#								
HEALTH INFORMATICS Balas (146)											
Johnston (171)											
Friedman (138)	#		#	#							
MEDICINE Altman (108)	#	#	#	#				#	#		
Chalmers 1990 (172)											
Chalmers 1981 (142)		#	~								
Cho (173)								#			
Colditz (174)											
Detsky (175)											
Evans (176)	#		#						#		
Goodman (143)	#	#	#			#					
Imperiale (177)											
Jadad (141)											
Kleijnen (178)											
Reisch (179)									~	#	#
Verhagen (180)											

PRESENTATION (CONTINUED)	Is the manuscript concise	Were references correct	Were keywords included	Is there proper reporting of denominators	Is the title informative/correct	Is there a lab package	State investigator involvement/roles	Were quantitative results understandable	Was text understandable	State sources of research support
COMPUTER SCIENCE Basili 1986 (158)										
Basili 1999 (159)						#				
Boudreau (160)										
Brooks (161)										
Fenton (16)										
Host (162)										
Jarvenpaa (163)										
Jedlitschka (113)										
Juristo 2001 (152)										
Juristo 2004 (164)					#					
Kitchenham 2002 (122)				#	·					#
Kitchenham 2006 (165)			#		#					
Lott (166)										
Moher 1981 (100)										
Moher 1982 (80)										
Pfleeger (167-170)										
Sadler (123)										

Singer (114)											
Sjoberg (94)											
Weinberg (119)											
Wohlin (153)							#				
HEALTH INFORMATICS Balas (146)											
Johnston (171)											
Friedman (138)								#			#
MEDICINE Altman (108)		#		#	#						#
Chalmers 1990 (172)											
Chalmers 1981 (142)											#
Cho (173)											
Colditz (174)											
Detsky (175)											
Evans (176)	#	#		#	#						
Goodman (143)	#			#	#				#		
Imperiale (177)											
Jadad (141)											
Kleijnen (178)											
Reisch (179)					#					#	#
Verhagen (180)											

OTHER ISSUES	Is there restricted generalisability across constructs	Were consent, confidentiality, ethical issues addressed adequately	Avoid experiment affecting overall industrial project environment	Was the relationship between industrial project and study defined	Was the experiment overly constrained	Was cost-effectiveness discussed	Were formative and summative studies performed	Were lab and field studies performed	Did the study go beyond the developer's point of view	Was feedback given to participants	Avoid preconceived opinion about treatment superiority	Is the study visible to researchers or practitioners
COMPUTER SCIENCE Basili 1986 (158)												#
Basili 1999 (159)												
Boudreau (160)												
Brooks (161)												
Fenton (16)												
Host (162)˭				~								
Jarvenpaa (163)												
Jedlitschka (113)		#				#						
Juristo 2001 (152)												
Juristo 2004 (164)												
Kitchenham 2002 (122)												
Kitchenham 2006 (165)												
Lott (166)		#									#	
Moher 1981 (100)												
Moher 1982 (80)												

Pfleeger (167-170)												
Sadler (123)				#	#							
Singer (114)												
Sjoberg (94)		#									#	
Weinberg (119)						#						
Wohlin (153)	#	#	#								#	
HEALTH INFORMATICS Balas (146)												
Johnston (171)												
Friedman (138)		#			#		#	#	#	#		
MEDICINE Altman (108)		#					#					
Chalmers 1990 (172)												
Chalmers 1981 (142)												
Cho (173)		#										
Colditz (174)												
Detsky (175)												
Evans (176)		#										#
Goodman (143)												
Imperiale (177)												
Jadad (141)												
Kleijnen (178)												
Reisch (179)		#					#					
Verhagen (180)												

Appendix B

2. How clear is the computing technology/method? *What is it? What does it do?*
|0 unclear| |1| |2| |3 moderately clear| |4| |5| |6 clear|

3. How clear is the benefit of the computing technology/method? *How is it important? How is it useful?*
|0 unclear| |1| |2| |3 moderately clear| |4| |5| |6 clear|

4. How clear are the objectives of the experiment?
|0 unclear| |1| |2| |3 moderately clear| |4| |5| |6 clear|

8. How clear is the independent variable(s)?
|0 unclear| |1| |2| |3 moderately clear| |4| |5| |6 clear|

9. How clear are the treatments (factor levels/alternatives)?
|0 unclear| |1| |2| |3 moderately clear| |4| |5| |6 clear|

11. How clear is the experimental site?
|0 unclear| |1| |2| |3 moderately clear| |4| |5| |6 clear|

12. How complete is the description of the schedule of the experiment?
|0 no description| |1 period length only e.g. 12 weeks| |2 partial date| |3 full date (d, m, y)|

14. Is it clear what the experimental unit is?
|0 unclear| |1| |2| |3 moderately clear| |4| |5| |6 clear|

20. Is it clear how treatment groups were formed? *How were subjects allocated to experimental groups e.g. random, nonrandom?*
|0 unclear| |1| |2| |3 moderately clear| |4| |5| |6 clear|

24. Are the materials representative of those that would be used in a real world setting? *If materials are unclear then NA.*
|0 not representative| |1| |2| |3 moderately representative| |4| |5| |6 representative| |-- NA|

25. If applicable, are the tasks required of the experimental unit clear?
|0 unclear| |1| |2| |3 moderately clear| |4| |5| |6 clear| |--NA|

26. If applicable, are the tasks representative of those that would be performed in a real-world setting? *If tasks are unclear then NA.*
|0 not representative| |1| |2| |3 moderately representative| |4| |5| |6 representative| |-- NA|

27. Are the outcomes clear?
|0 unclear| |1| |2| |3 moderately clear| |4| |5| |6 clear|

28. Are the outcomes justified?
|0 not justified| |1| |2| |3 moderately justified| |4| |5| |6 justified|

29. Are the data collection procedures clear e.g. instrumentation, actual procedure?
|0 unclear| |1| |2| |3 moderately clear| |4| |5| |6 clear|

33. For what percentage of main/primary outcomes was expected differences defined? *The expected difference is the pre-specified improvement in outcome from applying the technology/method.*
|0 0-25%| |1 26%-50%| |2 51%-75%| |3 76%-100%|

35. Are the investigators also the developers of the technology/method?
|0 yes| |1 no| |-- unknown or NA|

36. Did the developer of the technology/method financially support the investigators?
|0 yes| |1 no| |-- unknown or NA|

39. If applicable, do the investigators control for the checklist effect. *This occurs when subjects'
performance improves due to improved data collection rather than computations over that data e.g.
collecting well-structured inputs for a decision support system can improve outcomes rather than the system
itself. This can be quantified by having a control group that collects data but receives no system output e.g.
paper checklist.*
|0 not controlled or acknowledged| |1inadequate control| |2 controlled but effect not quantified| |3
effect quantified| |-- NA|

40. If applicable, do the investigators control for the data completeness effect? *This occurs when computer-
based data collection e.g. a log, is more complete than manual methods used by controls. This can be
avoided if data collection methods are the same for all groups.*
|0 not controlled or acknowledged| |1inadequate control| |2 controlled but effect not quantified| |3
effect quantified| |-- NA|

41. If applicable, do the investigators control for feedback effect? *Any form of performance feedback to
subjects (computerised or otherwise) can increase task performance. This can confound the effect of a
system on performance. To quantify the effect of a system over general feedback, a feedback-only control
group can be used.*
|0 not controlled or acknowledged| |1inadequate control| |2 controlled but effect not quantified| |3
effect quantified| |-- NA|

42. If applicable, do the investigators control for historical effects? *When experimental groups are assessed
at different times, other factors can arise between times to confound the results. This can be avoided by using
a parallel-group design.*
|0 not controlled or acknowledged| |1inadequate control| |2 controlled but effect not quantified| |3
effect quantified| |-- NA|

43. If experimental units are exposed to multiple treatments/variables, do the investigators control for the
interaction of different treatments/variables? *It may be difficult to distinguish results due to individual
treatment/variables or combinations.*
|0 not controlled or acknowledged| |1inadequate control| |2 controlled but effect not quantified| |3
effect quantified| |-- NA|

44. Are volunteer subjects used? *Volunteers tend to be systematically different to non-volunteers e.g. more
enthusiastic, informed etc.*
|0 yes| |1 no| |-- unknown|

45. What is the Hawthorne effect? *This occurs when subjects' performance improves due to investigator
scrutiny rather than the technology/method. This can be quantified by discreetly collecting data from a pre-
study control group.*
|0 not globally affecting control and treatment groups| |1 globally affecting control and treatment groups| |2
effect quantified|

52. If non-enrolment occurred, how adequate is the comparison of the non-enrolled to the enrolled? *Were
there systematic differences likely to affect outcomes? If it is unknown whether non-enrolment occurred then
NA. If there was full enrolment then NA.*
|0 inadequate| |1| |2| |3 moderately adequate| |4| |5| |6 adequate| |-- NA|

53. If there were losses/withdrawals, how adequate is the comparison of the lost/withdrawn to the enrolled? *Were there systematic differences likely to affect outcomes? If it is unknown whether there were losses/withdrawals then NA. If there were no losses/withdrawals then NA.*
|0 inadequate| |1| |2| |3 moderately adequate| |4| |5| |6 adequate| |-- NA|

54. If there were losses/withdrawals, how adequately are lost data handled in the statistical analysis? *If it is unknown whether there were losses/withdrawals then NA. If there were no losses/withdrawals then NA.*
|0 inadequate| |1| |2| |3 moderately adequate| |4| |5| |6 adequate| |--NA|

56. Are all hypotheses tested using inferential statistics?
|0 no| |1 partially| |2 yes|

58. Has manipulation of raw data e.g. handling of outliers, missing data, biased the results?
|0 strong bias| |1| |2| |3 moderately bias| |4| |5| |6 no bias|

62. Are too many tests used (and not corrected for)? *When applying too many tests, some may be significant due to chance. If corrected then answer 1.*
|0 yes| |1 no|

65. Was the person performing statistical analysis blinded?
|0 no or unknown| |1 yes|

66. Which statistical software package was used?
|0 not named| |1 name only| |2 name and version|

71. How adequate is the discussion on the practical importance of the findings?
|0 inadequate| |1| |2| |3 moderately adequate| |4| |5| |6 adequate|

72. For negative results, how adequate was the assessment of why? *E.g. due to type II error.*
|0 inadequate| |1| |2| |3 moderately adequate| |4| |5| |6 adequate| |-- NA|

74. Does the title indicate what the experiment was for and whether it was a controlled experiment? *E.g. controlled experiment of the effects of a decision support tool on productivity.*
|0 neither| |1 either| |2 both|

75. How accurate is the abstract in reporting the main content?
|0 inaccurate| |1| |2| |3 moderately accurate| |4| |5| |6 accurate|

76. Is the IMRAD (Introduction, Method, Results, and Discussion) style used?
|0 no| |1 partially| |2 yes|

77. Are graphics, figures and/or tables used appropriately e.g. understandable, labelled, accurately show the data etc?
|0 inappropriate||1| |2| |3 moderately appropriate| |4| |5| |6 appropriate|

78. Is the report complete? *Is there any further important information that should have been reported?*
|0 incomplete| |1| |2| |3 moderately complete| |4| |5| |6 complete|

79. Are details reported in inappropriate sections e.g. results in Introduction or Discussion rather than entirely in Results.
|0 yes| |1 no|

80. Is the report understandable?
|0 not understandable| |1| |2| |3 moderately understandable| |4| |5| |6 understandable|

Appendix C

STUDY	MICE-80 mean minus statistician item	MICE-80 mean with statistician item	MICE-38 mean minus statistician item	MICE-38 mean with statistician item	Statistician (1 = yes)	JIF	Authors	Pages	References	Year
Health informatics										
Bonevski (212)	0.634	0.635	0.608	0.610	1	2.39	6	9	70	1999
Brownbridge (213)	0.425	0.423	0.303	0.301	0		4	5	13	1986
Cannon (214)	0.534	0.532	0.388	0.385	0	3.979	2	8	26	2000
Christakis (215)	0.678	0.679	0.633	0.635	1	5.012	6	4	21	2001
Demakis (216)	0.642	0.643	0.631	0.633	1	23.175	9	6	26	2000
Dexter (217)	0.595	0.596	0.549	0.551	1	14.78	7	9	55	1998
Fitzmaurice (218)	0.408	0.410	0.331	0.335	1	1.938	5	3	17	1996
Fitzmaurice (219)	0.552	0.550	0.517	0.514	0	7.92	6	6	25	2000
Gonzalez (220)	0.581	0.580	0.502	0.499	0	1.518	4	7	22	1989
Hickling (221)	0.574	0.572	0.436	0.434	0	4.406	3	5	13	1989
Horn (222)	0.394	0.393	0.257	0.255	0	1.634	5	12	16	2002
Kuperman (223)	0.553	0.551	0.348	0.346	0	3.979	9	11	33	1999
Lewis (224)	0.572	0.570	0.523	0.521	0	1.558	4	7	28	1996
Lowensteyn (225)	0.585	0.587	0.592	0.595	1	2.39	6	8	21	1998
Mazzuca (226)	0.648	0.649	0.601	0.603	1	1.388	6	16	27	1990
McAllister (227)	0.697	0.698	0.663	0.665	1	9.245	5	5	22	1986
McDonald (228)	0.588	0.589	0.511	0.514	1	14.78	7	9	26	1984
Poller (229)	0.616	0.617	0.566	0.568	1	25.8	7	5	11	1998
Rosser (230)	0.577	0.576	0.501	0.498	0	6.862	3	7	30	1991
Rossi (231)	0.734	0.735	0.691	0.693	1	2.964	2	7	18	1997
Rotman (232)	0.722	0.723	0.642	0.644	1	3.979	10	9	20	1996
Ryff-de Leche (233)	0.538	0.536	0.449	0.447	0		5	9	14	1992
Schriger (234)	0.801	0.798	0.789	0.784	0	3.12	5	9	24	2001
Selker (235)	0.770	0.771	0.805	0.806	1	14.78	19	11	21	1998
Tamblyn (236)	0.759	0.760	0.759	0.760	1	6.862	8	8	50	2003
Tang (237)	0.519	0.517	0.404	0.402	0	3.979	4	7	25	1999
Thomas (238)	0.505	0.504	0.395	0.393	0	0.518	3	7	7	1983
Tierney (239)	0.607	0.605	0.521	0.518	0	23.175	4	10	30	1993
Vadher (240)	0.706	0.707	0.699	0.700	1	9.245	3	5	24	1997
Vadher (241)	0.557	0.556	0.493	0.490	0	0.921	3	5	13	1997
Verner (242)	0.549	0.548	0.410	0.408	0	2.029	8	5	28	1992
Wexler (243)	0.391	0.390	0.303	0.302	0		4	3	3	1975
Young (244)	0.386	0.384	0.272	0.271	0	0.551	1	5	5	1981
Computer science										
Alibabar (187)	0.627	0.626	0.600	0.598	0		2	9	27	2006
Alibabar (188)	0.653	0.651	0.605	0.601	0		3	10	46	2006
Anda (189)	0.522	0.521	0.453	0.451	0		2	11	23	2003
Arisholm (190)	0.499	0.500	0.531	0.534	1	1.03	3	47	19	2001
Briand (157)	0.622	0.620	0.571	0.568	0	2.132	3	18	29	2001

Bunse (191)	0.630	0.628	0.591	0.587	0	1.03	1	41	52	2006
Canfora (192)	0.624	0.622	0.629	0.626	0		5	8	15	2006
Golden (193)	0.534	0.532	0.430	0.428	0		3	10	16	2005
Hu (194)	0.411	0.410	0.356	0.354	0		4	8	36	2006
Johnson (195)	0.582	0.580	0.498	0.495	0		2	10	14	1997
Lopes (196)	0.441	0.440	0.316	0.314	0		3	10	11	1993
Lott (197)	0.604	0.602	0.590	0.587	0	1.03	1	21	14	1997
Muller (198)	0.571	0.570	0.562	0.559	0	0.592	1	14	27	2005
Myers (199)	0.529	0.530	0.438	0.439	0	1.509	1	9	11	1978
Myrtveit (156)	0.506	0.505	0.495	0.493	0	2.132	2	16	8	1999
Ng (200)	0.519	0.518	0.490	0.487	0		4	11	29	2006
Prechelt (201)	0.493	0.492	0.475	0.472	0	2.132	2	11	22	1998
Prechelt (202)	0.498	0.496	0.504	0.501	0	2.132	5	11	11	2001
Prechelt (203)	0.538	0.537	0.524	0.521	0	2.132	4	12	31	2002
Prechelt (204)	0.540	0.539	0.527	0.524	0	0.592	4	12	16	2003
Sears (205)	0.526	0.525	0.525	0.522	0		2	25	24	1994
Sonnenwald (206)	0.713	0.714	0.687	0.689	1		3	27	40	2003
Vokac (207)	0.555	0.554	0.606	0.603	0	1.03	5	47	19	2004
Wojcicki (208)	0.534	0.536	0.466	0.469	1		2	10	53	2006
Zettel (209)	0.601	0.599	0.600	0.596	0	1.03	1	28	47	2005

Appendix D

Item	Max Score	Albisser (291)	Augstein (292)	Col (293)	Davis (294)	Davison (295)	Emery (296)	Glassman (297)	Kaner (298)	Leibovici (299)	Martens (300)	Momtahan (289)	Montgomery (301)	Ozanne (302)	Peterson (303)	Protheroe (304)	Raebel (305)	Reeve (306)	Rothschild (290)	Schapira (307)	Taylor (308)	Thomson (309)
1	6	1	0	5	6	5	3	5	5	0	2	1	6	6	3	6	6	4	3	4	4	5
2	6	4	0	1	0	3	3	3	3	1	0	2	0	1	0	0	3	5	1	0	0	6
3	6	6	5	3	6	3	6	1	3	4	5	0	5	6	1	5	6	6	3	6	5	6
4	6	2	3	4	6	5	6	2	3	5	5	0	4	3	3	6	4	5	4	3	3	3
5	6	5	6	6	6	6	6	6	6	6	5	6	6	6	6	6	6	6	5	5	6	5
6	6	4	4	5	4	4	6	3	3	6	5	6	6	4	4	6	4	6	4	4	2	4
7	6	2	2	5	4	6	6	5	3	0	1	2	1	3	0	6	6	4	2	6	6	6
8	6	6	6	6	4	6	6	0	1	0	6	1	6	6	5	6	6	1	3	6	6	6
9	6	6	6	6	4	1	0	0	0	0	0	0	6	6	1	6	0	4	3	3	0	6
10	6	0	3	4	6	5	6	0	0	6	6	5	3	0	0	6	1	6	2	4	6	0
11	6	5	6	5	4	6	6	5	6	6	4	5	6	4	5	6	5	6	4	5	5	5
12	1	1	1	1	0	1	0	0	1	0	0	0	0	1	0	0	1	1	1	1	0	1
13	1	0	0	1	1	0	1	0	0	0	0	0	1	0	0	1	0	0	0	1	1	1
14	6	6	3	4	4	3	3	3	4	1	6	3	4	4	2	4	6	6	3	5	6	5
15	6	3	6	4	0	6	0	2	6	0	2	0	4	4	0	5	2	4	6	5	5	4
16	6	5	6	4	5	5	3	4	6	3	5	1	4	4	3	5	2	3	5	5	5	5
17	3	3	3	0	0	0	0	0	0	0	0	2	0	1	1	0	0	3	2	0	0	0
18	6	6	5	4	4	6	6	6	4	0	3	0	5	6	0	4	5	5	5	6	6	6
19	3	2	2		1		2		2	2	0	0		0				3	3	2	1	2
20	3	0	0		2		2	0		2	2	0		0	0		0		0		0	
21	2	1	0	0	1	0	0	0	0	0	2	0	0	0	0	0	2	0	0	0	2	0
22	2	0	2	0	0		0	2	0	2	0	0	0	0	0	0	2	1	2	0	2	0
23	6	6	6	6	5	6	6	6	3	0	4	0	6	6	0	6	5	3	5	6	6	6
24	6	5	6	6	6	1	6	6	6	4	6	0	6	4	3	3	5	5	3	5	6	6
25	6	0	3	6	6	0	6	6	6	5	6	0	6	0	0	5	0	5	0	5	5	6
26	6	3	6	6	6	6	6	4	4	1	5	1	6	4	2	5	6	5	6	6	3	6
27	3	3	3	1	3	3	3	3	3	0	1	0	2	3	0	2	3	3	3	3	3	1
28	2	2	2	1	2	2	2	2	0	0	2	0	2	1	0	2	0	2	0	1	2	2
29	6	6	6	6	6	5	6	6	6	6	6	6	6	6	6	6	6	6	6	6	6	6
30	6	6	6	6	6	6	6	5	6	0	6	0	6	4	5	3	5	3	5	5	6	5
31	1	0	0	1	1	1	1	1	0	0	1	0	0	0	0	0	1	0	1	1	1	0
32	1	0	0	1	1	1	1	1	0	0	1	0	0	0	0	0	1	0	1	1	1	0
33	1	0	0	1	1	0	1	1	1	0	1	0	0	1	0	0	0	0	1	0	0	1
34	6	2	2	6	6	4	6	1	2	2	2	0	3	2	1	6	2	4	6	4	6	2
35	6	1	2	6	4	4	3	1	1	0	2	0	3	1	0	6	2	4	5	4	3	1
36	6	3	3	5	6	6	5	6	6	0	6	4	6	6	1	6	4	6	5	6	5	6
37	6	3	3	6	6	5	4	5	6	3	6	1	3	3	2	6	2	2	5	6	6	5
38	6	2	2	4	6	5	4	3	4	0	4	1	4	3	2	6	3	3	6	5	6	5
Sum		110	119	135	140	125	137	103	107	66	120	43	129	107	55	146	115	127	116	134	134	134
Applicable		179	179	173	179	171	179	176	176	179	179	179	173	176	179	173	176	176	179	176	176	176

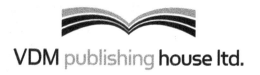

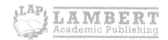
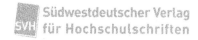

www.ingramcontent.com/pod-product-compliance
Lightning Source LLC
La Vergne TN
LVHW042333060326
832902LV00006B/143